Transhumanism and Transcendence

D1706404

Transhumanism and Transcendence

Christian Hope in an Age of Technological Enhancement

RONALD COLE-TURNER • *Editor*

GEORGETOWN UNIVERSITY PRESS | WASHINGTON, DC

Library of Congress Cataloging-in-Publication Data

   Transhumanism and transcendence : Christian hope in an age of technological enhancement /
  Ronald Cole-Turner, editor.
     p.   cm.
  Includes bibliographical references and index.
  ISBN 978-1-58901-780-1 (pbk. : alk. paper)
   1. Human body—Religious aspects—Christianity. 2. Theological anthropology—Christianity. 3. Technology—Religious aspects—Christianity. 4. Biotechnology—Religious aspects—Christianity. 5. Medical technology. Cole-Turner, Ronald, 1948–
  BT741.3.T73 2011
  261.5'6—dc22   2011013094

♾ This book is printed on acid-free paper meeting the requirements of the American National Standard for Permanence in Paper for Printed Library Materials.

15 14 13 12 11   9 8 7 6 5 4 3 2 First printing

Printed in the United States of America

To my parents

Contents

Chapter One

Introduction:
The Transhumanist Challenge

RONALD COLE-TURNER

Technology is being used more and more today in an attempt to enhance human lives by directly modifying human traits or capacities. Athletes use drugs to increase their strength or stamina. Cosmetic surgery is widely used around the world to improve physical appearance, while millions of men take drugs like Viagra to enhance their sexual performance. University students take prescription drugs not just to treat learning difficulties but to enhance their mental abilities. Others take drugs designed to treat anxiety and depression in order to elevate or brighten their mood.

The common feature here is the use of technology for the purpose of enhancement. As these technologies become more powerful and prevalent, a new challenge arises for theology, which is taken up by various Christian theologians and ethicists in the pages that follow. Today's technologies of human enhancement are largely limited to prescription drugs and surgery. Research is under way, however, on new and exotic technologies such as nanotechnology, information technology, cell regeneration, and implantable devices that interact directly with the brain. Any one of these fields may lead to far more powerful ways to expand human powers, augment human capacities, and—arguably at least—enhance human lives.

But what exactly is meant by enhancement? According to Maxwell J. Mehlman, "a biomedical enhancement . . . raises a person up by improving performance, appearance, or capability. If only it were that simple."[1] Any attempt to define enhancement raises new questions that are anything but easy to answer. For example, there seems to be no way to define enhancement without saying that it is an increase in worth or an improvement. But how do we define "improvement" or, as Mehlman puts it, that which "raises a person up"? The athlete may think that being stronger is a clear enhancement, but not if it comes at the cost of overall health. Smarter is better, unless of course it leads to memories that cannot be escaped or softened with time. Who really is in a position to say what counts as an improvement or an enhancement—who, that is, except the person who is modified? "For the most part," Mehlman writes, "an enhancement is an improvement if the enhanced person thinks it is one."[2]

The judgment about whether a technological modification really enhances is left to the "enhanced person." This is probably the only way a society like ours can settle what would otherwise be endless debates about what we value most and what it takes to increase or improve what we value. After all, we leave it to each individual to decide the meaning of a good life, allowing each person to choose from all the competing versions of a life well lived. If enhancing our lives means increasing its value or goodness, something defined only by personal choice, then what counts as an enhancement can only be judged for and by each individual.

But even if we leave it to the individual to decide what counts as an enhancement, other perplexing questions about enhancement still arise. Are individuals really free to choose their view of life or their way of achieving and enhancing that good? Does it matter if they are coerced into using enhancement technology, either overtly or covertly, for instance by an employer that wants them to be more productive? And if they are free of coercion, can society as a whole really trust every adult to make prudent decisions? Perhaps limits must be put in place to keep people from enhancing the very traits that others find offensive or dangerous. And we must also ask: How far can an individual be changed without becoming someone different, even "someone else"? (For more on this point, see chapter 12 in this book.) And above all, how far can humanity be modified without becoming "posthuman"?

With questions like these, it should come as no surprise that ours is an age not just of expanding technologies but also of growing debates about the ethics of these technologies. What may be surprising, however, is that relatively few religious scholars and leaders have joined in, despite the fact that the religious themes are often apparent at the very surface of these debates. Theological explorations of human enhancement through technology or on the subject of transhumanism are just beginning to appear.[3]

This volume includes chapters by many of the key contributors to the theological discussion so far. Our goal is to contribute to the public understanding of the role that theology might play in the debate about transhumanism and the use of technologies of human enhancement, to clarify the challenge brought by technology and transhumanism to theology, and to explore as far as possible some of the forms of human yearning for transcendence that are found in theology and transhumanism. The present chapter introduces transhumanism and suggests some of the ways in which it raises questions for all human beings, especially for Christians interested in theology. The next chapters explore some of the historical antecedents of transhumanism, whereas the midsection of the book asks what insight theology might bring to some of the bioethical reflection about technology and transhumanist visions. The final chapters address the theological challenge that is posed by enhancement technology and especially by the transhumanist vision, arguing sometimes at odds with each other about the most appropriate theological response. Our first task, however, is to try to define enhancement and consider how it differs from therapy.

Therapy versus Enhancement

Defining enhancement by distinguishing it from therapy seems obvious, almost intuitive. It is one thing to treat a disease or to repair an injury and quite another to use the very same techniques to help someone become unusually strong or beautiful. According to Mehlman, "by definition enhancements are not aimed at preventing, treating, or mitigating the effects of a disease or disorder."[4] Medical insurance companies agree by denying all claims for "cosmetic" surgery. In fact, if we are going to address the topic of enhancement at all, we find ourselves drawing the therapy/enhancement distinction in order to limit the scope of the subject matter before us. And so it is that in almost every discussion of enhancement technology, the subject matter is defined as the use of technology, especially medicine, to "treat" or modify human beings quite apart from any disease. For example, cognitive enhancement occurs when those without any diagnosis use drugs that may have been developed and approved to treat cognitive impairment but that are now being used solely to boost brain power.

Drawing the distinction between therapy and enhancement may be intuitive and unavoidable, but it is important that we not expect too much from the distinction. For example, sometimes critics of enhancement technology use the distinction not to identify a topic for discussion but to brand the whole attempt as immoral. They recognize that the same biomedical technology may be used for therapy and enhancement, and, not wishing to condemn this technology altogether, insist that a clear line can be drawn between the moral use of this technology for therapy and its immoral use for enhancement. The problem, of course, is that the line between therapy and enhancement may seem obvious, but it is anything but clear. "Disease" itself is a socially constructed category, not something unambiguous in nature, and the list of diseases changes over time, often in light of cultural preferences or the marketing of a new drug. If "therapy" treats "disease," it treats a moving target. Furthermore, sometimes individuals treated for a disease are helped so much that they become healthier than "normal," however the human "normal" is defined at various stages of life. In the course of one medical treatment, they experience therapy that brings them up to normal health and enhancement that takes them beyond.

Leon Kass, the former chair of the President's Council on Bioethics and certainly no friend of technological enhancement, is right when he concludes: "Those who introduced this distinction [between therapy and enhancement] hoped by this means to distinguish between the acceptable and the dubious or unacceptable uses of biomedical technology: therapy is always ethically fine, enhancement is, at least prima facie, ethically suspect."[5] He continues: "But this distinction is inadequate and finally unhelpful to the moral analysis."[6] And then he redirects our attention away from attempts to draw a morally significant distinction between therapy and enhancement and back to the central question posed by the use of technology in the first place: "Needless arguments about whether or not something is or is not an 'enhancement' get in the way of the proper question: What are the good and bad uses of biotechnical power? What makes a use 'good,' or even just 'acceptable'?"[7]

The therapy/enhancement distinction will not go away, nor should it, but its value is limited. Above all it should not seduce us into thinking that we can draw simple lines that separate the good and bad uses of technology. The power of technology to transform humanity raises questions and concerns that go far beyond any definitions or boundaries we might draw around therapy, and as Kass suggests, it is to these wider questions that we must turn our attention.

Embracing Technology

A central issue in the debate is the issue of the proper role of technology. After all, almost no one objects to the idea that human beings should strive to enhance or improve themselves. The desirability of human enhancement is the presupposition underlying most of our attitudes about the duties of parents, the value of education, and the need for that hard work that prepares us for life. And to say that religion, Christianity in particular, also endorses at least some form of human enhancement is an understatement in the extreme.

At the very core of Christianity is the dynamic of human redemption and transformation. Christian theology grounds this transformation in its distinctive view of God, who enters the human condition in order to transform it. An interesting comparison can be found between two distinctions, one made in theology and the other in bioethics. The distinction in theology is between redemption and glorification, between God redeeming humanity by restoring us to an original state from which we have fallen and glorifying or transforming us far above any original status. The bioethics distinction that is similar, and perhaps related historically, is of course the one between therapy and enhancement. Redemption and therapy are both aimed at restoring what was (or what should be regarded as a "normal" state, even if it never actually existed), whereas glorification and enhancement take us far beyond toward something completely new. In both cases, those who argue for the legitimacy of therapy/redemption (but not enhancement/glorification), whether secular or religious, seem to presuppose a definition of normal grounded either in a creationist theology or some secular alternative that views the human species, if not as static, then as having attained a status that no one should dare to alter without threatening all that humans hold dear.

The main point, however, is that human transformation is central to Christian thought, and thus it affects the way in which Christian theology understands not just the character but the very being of God as triune and as capable of entering into and taking up the human condition, thereby transforming it beyond all human expectation. This belief is summed up in the simple saying that God becomes like us so that we might be made like God. This saying goes back at least to Irenaeus of Lyon, who died in about 200 CE, and it has been echoed by major theologians ever since. Vladimir Lossky restates the saying and comments on its significance:

> "God made Himself man, that man might become God." These
> powerful words, which we find for the first time in St. Irenaeus, are again
> found in the writings of St. Athanasius, St. Gregory of Nazianzus, and St.
> Gregory of Nyssa. The Fathers and Orthodox theologians have repeated
> them in every century with the same emphasis, wishing to sum up in this
> striking sentence the very essence of Christianity: an ineffable descent
> of God to the ultimate limit of our fallen condition, even unto death—a
> descent of God which opens to men a path of ascent, the unlimited
> vistas of the union of created beings with the Divinity.[8]

The significance of this saying for our purposes in this volume is that it shows the centrality and depth of the theme of human transformation in Christianity. Through the centuries and continuing today, Christians have debated how far it is possible for human beings to be improved, and even more sharply about whether it is possible for us to improve ourselves or whether such improvement (or more precisely, redemption and sanctification) is utterly by grace acting without the cooperation or joint action of the one who is being redeemed. But there has been almost no debate at all about the need for the improvement of human beings.

Human enhancement through technology, however, is another question. Even when the goal is the same—smarter children, for example, or more loving and faithful spouses—the method that is used seems to matter a great deal. Nearly everyone is more comfortable with the idea that we improve our cognitive ability through the mental disciplines of traditional education rather than through the use of technological "shortcuts." Even our choice of technology seems to matter: We are more at peace with using a calculator or software that checks our spelling than with taking a pill that makes us concentrate more clearly so that we can solve more demanding problems in arithmetic.

Some who prefer "old-fashioned hard work" might object that the use of technology is a kind of cheating, as if technology makes achievement effortless and therefore "fake" or illegitimate, something gained but not earned. Others counter that technology of some kind or other is an inescapable part of being human. If calculators are a kind of cheating, why is it legitimate to enhance human ability by using a much earlier technology called paper? If computer implants trouble us because they might put a library of data in the brain, how do we justify books and libraries buildings, which are also data-access technologies that enhance our cognitive abilities? Is there not something profoundly and essentially human about creating technologies that enhance what we most value? Is it not part of our nature to invent, to enhance our powers, and to set new expectations for striving and achieving? Is not our nature as a species shaped by evolutionary processes in which tens of millions of years of tool making has played a selective role? But if so, does it matter how far we go, especially in putting these technologies inside us in such a way that we no longer experience the joy of "going" to the library but rather experience implanted memory as indistinguishable from "natural" memory? And so the debate goes on.

For secular bioethics the question of the proper role of technology in human enhancement is usually explored in the context of the philosophy of technology that emerged in the Enlightenment, most notably in the work of Francis Bacon, through to the various critics of technology, especially those grounded in the work of Martin Heidegger or Hans Jonas. For Christian theology, however, the question of technology draws upon all these sources but fits more properly within the larger theological question of the meaning of humanity as created in the image of God, living always in need of redemptive grace, and destined in Jesus Christ for transformation and everlasting life. How does Christianity understand technology—particularly its growing powers to transform human beings—within the framework of this theological vision? It is no longer possible, if indeed it ever was, to see technology as irrelevant to the theological meaning of humanity. One way or another, the transformations through technology are part of the larger cosmic drama of creation and redemption. But should we think of technology as a misguided effort to save ourselves, a refusal to live as God intends and await the salvation God brings? Or is it a risky but necessary way in which we open ourselves to what God is doing in us and through us, thereby allowing God's work to be done in us and through us by new means?

Identity and Authenticity: Enhancing the Individual

When we use technology for enhancement, we change more than just our bodies or our biochemistry or our performance. We are embodied creatures, and any use of technology that affects any part affects the whole being, including the very core of identity and personality, our mental powers of memory, understanding, and will, what traditionally has been called the soul. In some respects, all technology transforms those who use it or upon whom it is applied. Technology that is pointed at what surrounds the human organism affects the organism indirectly but often profoundly. Technological changes to our environment rebound in changes in ourselves, something that has been true at the species level in the history of our evolution but is also true on the individual level, in our own adjustment to the changing world around us.

More than that, our use of technology changes the way we see the world around us. No longer does it appear as given and unchangeable but more like a tentative proposal that we can accept or change at our discretion. Likewise, when technology is now turned inward upon ourselves, on our bodies and brains, we are changed more directly, more intentionally, and in the end more profoundly than ever before. Furthermore, just as technology aimed at the world around us inclines us to see nature as something to be changed, so technology turned on ourselves will teach us to see ourselves in a new way, as our own projects for improvement. The aim of the technologies of human enhancement is not to change the world but to change ourselves to fit better, to compete better, or to live better in the world as it is. And along the way, these technologies change the way we see ourselves, turning our bodies and brains into something to be changed at will.

The paradox, of course, is that the will is changed in the process. It may have made sense once to say something like this: "I will use technology to change the world around me. I will decide what changes to make, and I will remain largely unaltered over the course of the changes, the sovereign agent who judges the actions." But now, as we turn technology on ourselves so that we change our own bodies and brains, the "I" is swept up in the change and modified through its own action. When these technologies of human enhancement get inside us, they become part of us, turning us into our own products and blurring the lines we once drew between subject and object, agent and effect. When "I" use technology to change myself, just who is this "I" who decides and who is the "I" that is the result of the decision? Have I tried to draw an untenable line between the self that chooses and the self that is chosen, between self will and willed self?

Through technology, it is possible today to modify the memory in limited ways. In the future biomedical technology might offer powerful tools to increase or diminish the storing of memories. Unpleasant or traumatic memories can be selectively deleted. (For more on eliminating memory and emotion, see chapter 10.) The memory of what is about to be experienced or learned can be intensified, and the general capacity and acuity of memory can be heightened, if only to combat the effects of aging, or at least these are the hopes of researchers in the field. Not just memory, however, but psychological mood can be modified. More difficult but not impossible is the modification of our moral predispositions, our attachment or bond to other human beings (e.g., our spouse), and our level of self-esteem. The pathway of these modifications is through the biochemistry of the brain, but the capacities or traits that are modified lie at the very core of personal identity, affecting the deepest desires of the heart and the hidden motivations of the will.

How are we to think of the self that modifies itself? Is one real and the other fake or inauthentic? Assuming that there is not some changeless core of the soul that is immune to the transformations of the body and brain, some immaterial self that is untouched and unchanged by these neurological interventions, how are we to think of the human person as a continuous identity through change, especially change that is elected and effected and then serves as the basis for yet more technologically managed changes? Some see this as a kind of suicide whereby the old self wills its end by using technology to become someone else. For example, Susan Schneider writes: "For even if you would like to become 'superintelligent,' knowingly embarking upon a path that trades away one or more of your essential properties would be tantamount to suicide—that is, to your intentionally causing yourself to cease to exist."[9]

This conundrum is hardly new for Christian theology. Paul's theology is full of the paradox of transforming grace, whereby the "old self" is put to death and the "new self," the new identity of the Christian "in Christ," comes into existence, yet without the disappearance of the old body or the total negation of the old behavior, at least not until the final resurrection. Paul writes: "I have been crucified with Christ; and it is no longer I who live, but it is Christ who lives in me" (Gal 2:19–20). In this important text Paul is quite explicit about the paradox of the personal identity of the Christian, whose old self is being transformed into a new self, at once more real and authentic and yet profoundly different from the original self. For Paul and for Christianity, the identity of the new self is not grounded in the wishes of the old self, as is the case for the advocates of the uses of the technologies of human enhancement. Rather, the new self is the gradual creation of the *persona* of Christ ("it is Christ who lives in me") at the expense of the desires of the old self, which is diminished rather than enhanced. Christianity and transhumanism share the notion that the self is being transformed to the point where it will no longer be the same self. But Christianity and transhumanism could not be more different in how they view the goal of transformation. For Christianity, it is to put the old self to death in order to be like Christ in his resurrection and glorification; for transhumanism and for the advocates of technological enhancement, the goal is to bring the old self to a higher life while worrying about whether it will remain the same.

If the paradox of personal transformation is nothing new for Christian theology, the possibility of technology as the means of such transformation is both novel and perplexing. If Christians believe it is God's will for them to be more committed to their marriage partners, and a pill seems to make this possible, is it God's will to cause this change through a pill? Julian Savulescu and Anders Sandberg believe that technology should be used to increase romantic attachment: "Love is one of the fundamental aspects of human existence. It is to a large part biologically determined. We should use our growing knowledge of the neuroscience of love to enhance the quality of love by biological manipulation."[10] Should Christians agree?

Saying no seems wrong in light of all the ways in which Christians use medical technology, not only believing it is God's will but also praying that it will be effective. Saying yes seems odd because it seems to undercut or at least to reroute what Christians say they believe about the power of God to make us, if not perfectly holy, then at least morally better human beings. We could say that God does this in part through technology, just as we have always said that God does this in part through the church, our parents, or the influence of friends. Is this simply a case of Christians needing to update their repertoire of the modalities of grace? And might we blunt the scope of the updating by saying that there are always aspects of ourselves—the deepest sins and the predisposition toward sinning that lurks inside us, and above all our longing for oneness with the divine—that technology in principle will never touch, so use it in its limited ways without fear? Others will argue that grace and technology cannot work together precisely because technology is so much within our control and therefore always a threat and never an aid to grace.

When secular bioethics leaves it up to the individual to decide whether any particular technological modification really enhances, it opens itself to an interesting problem, one not faced in at least the same way by Christian theology. What are we to think if, after the technological enhancement, there is a change of mind—literally? Before the modification, the person completely understands and truly believes that the change is an enhancement. After the modification, the person completely understands and truly believes that it is not an enhancement, not because anything went wrong but because the enhancement worked and the moral core of the person has been changed. In such a case, is the change an enhancement? If all we can do is to leave the choice to the person, to which person are we leaving it? For Christian theology, however, if technology is used at all, its role is not to satisfy the will, either before or after the change, but to transform the person in the direction of the new creation in Jesus Christ, a theme that is explored more fully in the final chapter of this book.

Beyond the Human Species: The Challenge of Transhumanism

The technologies of human enhancement raise a puzzling question about the transformation of the human individual: Is the enhanced person still the same person? They raise an even more profound question, however, about the transformation of the human species: Is the enhanced person still human? At what point if ever will technology produce a change that results in the emergence of a new species beyond *Homo sapiens*? Some believe that given enough time, technology will modify human beings so much that they will no longer be human in the usual sense but will have become some other species of hominid. If this were to happen, would it amount to a kind of species suicide, the death of human nature as evolved and as we have always known it? And if so, would this be a step of technologically sophisticated lunacy, something akin, say, to a mass exchange of nuclear weapons? Or is there something deep in evolution itself that drives us forward in this direction so that we would have to regard such a step as comparable to the evolution of conscious or self-conscious beings?

Questions like these lie at the heart of the debate over transhumanism. Transhumanists see human nature as incomplete, human biology as limiting, and human technology as the pathway to a new form of humanity. Critics see this as a kind of mass death, a willful destruction of humanity. Theologians, as we will see in the subsequent chapters of this book, are suspicious of the optimism and the pretensions of transhumanists but divided in their opinion about transhumanism's core claim that human beings should use technology to enhance human nature.

What is transhumanism? In the simplest terms, it is a movement that advocates the development and use of new technologies to improve human capacities and enhance human lives. According to James J. Hughes, transhumanism holds to "the proposition that human beings should use technology to transcend the limitations of the body and brain."[11] Nick Bostrom defines transhumanism this way: "Transhumanism is a loosely defined movement that has developed gradually over the past two decades, and can be viewed as an outgrowth of secular humanism and the Enlightenment. It holds that current human nature is improvable through the use of applied science and other rational methods, which may make it possible to increase human health-span, extend our intellectual and physical capacities, and give us increased control over our own mental states and moods."[12]

A more lengthy definition is provided in "The Transhumanist FAQ" posted on the Internet by Nick Bostrom, according to which transhumanism is

1. The intellectual and cultural movement that affirms the possibility and desirability of fundamentally improving the human condition through applied reason, especially by developing and making widely available technologies to eliminate aging and to greatly enhance human intellectual, physical, and psychological capacities.
2. The study of the ramifications, promises, and potential dangers of technologies that will enable us to overcome fundamental human limitations, and the related study of the ethical matters involved in developing and using such technologies.[13]

The common theme that runs through these definitions is that human biology should be modified by technology, even to the point of fundamental or species change.

Transhumanists advocate the use of technology to change the human species, but in what direction or with what goal in mind? Bioethics leaves the question of what counts as a personal enhancement up to the individual. Accordingly, transhumanists today leave the question of species enhancement up to the aggregate of individual choices made by those with the means and the motivation to use the emerging technologies of enhancement. There appears to be no invisible hand guiding the process, no deep purpose or goal of evolution, and no objective measure of progress along the pathway of species enhancement.

This is not how Julian Huxley or Pierre Teilhard de Chardin, however, used the word "transhumanism" in the 1950s. Teilhard was a Jesuit priest also trained in paleontology, and some of his ideas are explored briefly in chapters 2 and 3. His theological transhumanism, centered on a controversial vision of the future of Christian hope achieved through future human evolution, landed him in a great deal of trouble during his lifetime. Huxley, who though an agnostic was close to Teilhard, introduced the term "transhumanism" this way in 1957: "The human species can, if it wishes, transcend itself—not just sporadically, an individual here in one way, an individual there in another way, but in its entirety, as humanity. We need a name for this new belief. Perhaps transhumanism will serve: man remaining man, but transcending himself, by realizing new possibilities of and for his human nature."[14] Huxley goes on to identify himself as a believer in transhumanism, adding that "once there are enough people who can truly say that, the human species will be on the threshold of a new kind of existence, as different from ours as ours is from that of Pekin man. It will at last be consciously fulfilling its real destiny."[15] Huxley seems to suggest that technology will create a new species of hominid, more advanced than its Creator.

For Huxley and Teilhard, transhumanism is not simply a proposition or a cultural movement. It is the future of evolution itself, grounded in objective reality quite apart from human awareness but now known to us through the science of evolution, which is being driven forward not just by genetic mutation and natural selection but also by technology aimed at transcending the evolved form of the human species.

Fading echoes of this "future of evolution" claim can be found in the thought of today's transhumanists. For example, according to Bostrom, "Transhumanists view human nature as a work-in-progress, a half-baked beginning that we can learn to remold in desirable ways. Current humanity need not be the endpoint of evolution. Transhumanists hope that by responsible use of science, technology, and other rational means we shall eventually manage to become posthuman, beings with vastly greater capacities than present human beings have."[16] But it is instructive to look carefully at statements like the "Transhumanist Declaration," where we read: "Humanity will be radically changed by technology in the future. We foresee the feasibility of redesigning the human condition, including such parameters as the inevitability of aging, limitations on human and artificial intellects, unchosen psychology, suffering, and our confinement to the planet earth."[17] The change may be radical, even species-altering. But the goal is defined by getting rid of what we do not like, not by the deep logic of the evolutionary process. In a similar way, Bostrom is candid about what counts as "progress." Progress for today's transhumanist is not the evolutionary advancement of biology but our expanded freedom from biology: "To a transhumanist, progress occurs when more people become more able to shape themselves, their lives, and the ways they relate to others, in accordance with their own deepest values."[18]

According to transhumanism, the final result of the technological modification of human nature is not something "better," merely something different, something no longer human, something we might call "posthuman." The word "posthuman," however, is somewhat confusing because it has been used recently in a quite different context where it has been given a far different meaning, not primarily associated with technology and transhumanism but with some of the cultural and literary movements of the past generation. In fact, transhumanists like Bostrom seem wary of the word "posthuman" because of its literary use. He defines posthumans as "possible future beings whose basic capacities so radically exceed those of present humans as to be no longer unambiguously human by our current standards."[19] He clearly wants to dissociate the transhumanist's use of "posthuman" from its literary meaning, arguing that literary posthumanism is a change of consciousness while transhumanism is a change of biology through technology. "Some authors write as though simply by changing our self-conception, we have become or could become posthuman. This is a confusion or corruption of the original meaning of the term. The changes required to make us posthuman are too profound to be achievable by merely altering some aspect of psychological theory or the way we think about ourselves. Radical technological modifications to our brains and bodies are needed."[20] But then he pleads a kind of agnosticism, saying that the changes expected from technology are so great that the consequences cannot be predicted. He writes: "Posthumans might shape themselves and their environment in so many new and profound ways that speculations about the detailed features of posthumans and the posthuman world are likely to fail."[21]

The difference between the transhumanist and the literary views of posthumanism is intriguing and deserves the sort of attention given it in chapter 8 of this book. The now-classic statement of what we are calling "literary posthumanism" is found in N. Katherine Hayles's *How We Became Posthuman*. According to Thomas Carlson, Hayles "defines the posthuman very clearly and concretely by its contrast with the logic that defines the subject of modern Western liberal humanism. If the latter is understood as a discrete, self-possessed, and self-governing individual, who exists as such 'by nature' and thus prior to the involvements of social being and its prosthetic supports, the posthuman subject is instead an indeterminate, irreducibly relational, and endlessly adaptive figure whose intelligence and agency are not simply possessed or controlled by the individual or his will, but always already distributed throughout complex networks that exceed, even as they constitute, any individual."[22] In contrast to Hayles and Carlson, the posthuman that lies ahead for transhumanism is not just a continuation of the self-governing individual but the individual set free of anything biological that interferes with this governing.

Technology and Transhumanism: A New Challenge for Theology

It may seem tempting to many to respond to transhumanism by ignoring or dismissing it. After all, as a cultural movement, it claims only a few thousand members, hardly the critical mass needed to launch the next stage of human evolution. But ignoring transhumanism comes at the risk of failing to see the more basic and pervasive dynamic upon which it depends. Even if all the dues-paying transhumanists go away, the technology of human enhancement is here not just to stay but to work its transformations. Of course, it is possible to focus our attention on technological enhancement without discussing transhumanism. Mehlman's *The Price of Perfection* contains no references to transhumanism in its index. A recent report by the British Medical Association on cognitive enhancement offers this assessment: "Philosophers speculate about the possibility and the implications of people becoming 'post-human' or 'trans-human' and our development into a new species that has 'super-human' powers. But this should not distract us from the very real and practical issues that are confronting us now, or will confront us in the near future."[23]

Of course there are some "very real and practical issues" that are complex and require careful thought. But to suggest that it is a distraction to consider the broadest possible context of our actions is to give way to an even more dangerous distraction, one that focuses only on the challenge of the moment and fails to see the full context that shapes our attitudes and choices. In this regard transhumanism renders an invaluable service to humanity, for by suggesting that we are doing away with ourselves—and that this is a good thing—transhumanism is forcing us to ask uncomfortable questions about our deepest desires, the means we use to achieve them, and the final outcome of all our technological transformations.

The longings that lie at the core of transhumanism are familiar to anyone who knows the texts of nearly any of the world's religions or traditional philosophies. Our situation is new, not because human beings have begun for the first time to yearn for long or endless lives of perfect health and greater intellect, but because the development of recent technology seems to suggests that, even if these goals are not now achievable, they may become so, at least in part, in the decades or centuries that lie ahead. Transhumanism may exceed technology today, but the gap is closing. It is no longer just another fantasy.

Theology in particular is being challenged by transhumanism to address questions that are too easily set aside. Is there direction or purpose in evolution that is grounded in the creative purposes of God even if not wholly discernible by science, a future and a purpose that we human beings can now begin to comprehend and in which we can play a part, for instance through technology? How are we to regard nonhuman species and our role, intentional or not, in their modification? How are we to think about the deep human yearning for transcendence, the longing to go beyond what we are given as biological creatures and to enter into what we seem destined to become, whether by our own design and achievement or because there is a God who has made us for something beyond ourselves?

Questions like these are explored throughout this book. In chapter 2 Michael Burdett explores some of the predecessors of today's transhumanists, taking us first to the writings of Francis Bacon, whose religious convictions were clear to his contemporaries but which are often forgotten today when he is simply regarded as an exponent of empiricism and practical science, what we have come to know as technology. Burdett also introduces us to the writings of the Russian intellectual N. F. Fedorov, and then briefly to Pierre Teilhard de Chardin. In chapter 3 David Grummett explores the thought of Teilhard more deeply, tracing his influence on today's transhumanists while also showing how clearly rooted Teilhard was in Christian theology, even while expounding a less-than-official interpretation. Although other antecedents might be chosen, it is remarkable that these historical examples suggest that transhumanism, if not born of Christianity, is solidly grounded in traditional Christian visions of the future, secularized now through technology as the new pathway to what lies ahead.

In chapter 4 Karen Lebacqz draws our attention to the more explicitly bioethical themes of human dignity and whether transhumanism is its full expression or its worst violation. Do enhancement technologies threaten something essential about what makes us human, or are they the most eloquent affirmation of human creativity? Finding neither argument fully persuasive, Lebacqz sounds a note that runs through this volume: Christians may be hopeful about the use of technology but also cautious, mindful not just of biblical warnings but also of historical failures. Ted Peters takes us further into this question in chapter 5 by arguing that transhumanists are a bit naive in their optimism and their failure to see how technology can go wrong even when it goes right. Christians should be wary of transhumanism, Peters suggests, not because they are wedded to the status quo but because, ironically, only they seem prepared to recognize the degree of change that human beings truly need. Patching up our "half-baked" human nature will not solve the problem that lies at the core of our humanity.

Cyborgs take center stage in the next two chapters. In chapter 6 Stephen Garner argues that technologies that will enhance human beings will have the tendency to blur the boundaries (whether in nature or only in our mind) between the human and the nonhuman or between the living and the nonliving. When conceptual boundaries are blurred, people become apprehensive because, quite literally, they no longer know how to think about things. For Garner, however, the pathway forward is not to stop technology but to recognize that cybernetics (or more generally, "hybridity," the mixing of species or natures) is fundamental to Christianity, a way of unifying rather than confusing. In chapter 7 J. Jeanine Thweatt-Bates takes the discussion forward by drawing upon the idea of the "feminist cyborg," which is not some creation of technology so much as a recognition that women find that they inevitably step out of the boundaries created for them by modern Western thought. She explores this idea by criticizing its misuse by several transhumanists, thereby offering a critique of the tendency among transhumanists to view the human self as disembodied.

In chapter 8 Celia Deane-Drummond argues that the mistaken idea that human flourishing is to be found in freedom from the limitations of biology is rooted in a long-standing theological tendency to draw too sharp a line between human beings and other animals. Too often, theology drew a line by arguing the human beings are uniquely rational and that this point of uniqueness is the basis for our being in the image of God. In transhumanism, the idea reappears in the notion that humans will be enhanced through a form of rationality set free from biology.

In chapter 9 Todd Daly explores the similarities and differences between the transhumanist goal of extending the human lifespan and the Christian hope of eternal life, suggesting that Christian practices might have the effect of extending the life span but that the hope of the Christian lies not just in the length of life but also in its moral and spiritual character. In chapter 10 Michael Spezio endorses a theological perspective that is largely sympathetic to transhumanism and open to the enhancement of human strengths. On this basis, he argues against those who want to base human moral reasoning on strictly rational as opposed to emotional and relational grounds by eliminating some forms of human emotion and specific memories, such as the memory of traumatic events. For him, this is a loss of human capacity, not an enhancement.

In chapter 11 Brent Waters takes the view that though human frailties and limitations cannot be called good, they are nonetheless vindicated by the Incarnation of God in Jesus Christ, who assumes our condition and thereby already transcends it for us and in us, if only we will remain creaturely. In chapter 12 Gerald McKenny contrasts the transcendence sought by transhumanists and by Christians, arguing that Christians are wary of transhumanism not because they oppose going beyond the present but because they oppose going beyond the human. Finally, chapter 13 draws some of these themes together by asking about the meaning of salvation or religious transformation in an age of technological enhancement.

Notes

1. Mehlman, *Price of Perfection*, 6.
2. Ibid.
3. E.g., see Deane-Drummond and Scott, eds., *Future Perfect?*; and Waters, *This Mortal Flesh*.
4. Mehlman, *Perfection*, 8.
5. Kass, "Ageless Bodies, Happy Souls," 13.
6. Ibid.
7. Ibid. For more on the therapy/enhancement distinction, see chapter 12.
8. Lossky, *In the Image and Likeness of God*, 97.
9. Schneider, *Future Minds*.
10. Savulescu and Sandberg, "Neuroenhancement," 42.
11. Hughes, "Compatibility of Religious and Transhumanist Views." Cf. Hughes, *Citizen Cyborg*, 155.
12. Bostrom, "In Defense of Posthuman Dignity."
13. Bostrom, "Transhumanist FAQ 2.1," 5.
14. Huxley, "Transhumanism," 17.
15. Ibid.
16. Bostrom, "Transhumanist Values."
17. Transhumanist Association, "Transhumanist Declaration," 2002.
18. Bostrom, "Transhumanist FAQ 2.1," 5.
19. Ibid.
20. Ibid., 6.
21. Ibid.
22. Carlson, *Indiscrete Image*, 15.
23. British Medical Association, *Boosting Your Brainpower*, 2–3.

References

Bostrom, Nick. "In Defense of Posthuman Dignity." *Bioethics* 19 (2005): 202–14.
———. "The Transhumanist FAQ 2.1." www.transhumanism.org/resources/FAQv21.pdf.
———. "Transhumanist Values." www.nickbostrom.com/ethics/values.html.
British Medical Association. *Boosting Your Brainpower: Ethical Aspects of Cognitive Enhancements*. London: British Medical Association, 2007.
Carlson, Thomas H. *The Indiscrete Image: Infinitude and Creation of the Human*. Chicago: University of Chicago Press, 2008.

Deane-Drummond, Celia, and Peter M. Scott, eds. *Future Perfect? God, Medicine and Human Identity*. London: T. & T. Clark International, 2006.

Hayles, N. K. *How We Became Posthuman: Virtual Bodies in Cybernetics, Literature, and Informatics*. Chicago: University of Chicago Press, 1999.

Hughes, James J. *Citizen Cyborg: Why Democratic Societies Must Respond to the Redesigned Human of the Future*. Cambridge, MA: Westview Press, 2004.

———. "The Compatibility of Religious and Transhumanist Views." *Global Spiral*, 2007. www.metanexus.net/magazine/tabid/68/id/9930/Default.aspx.

Huxley, Julian. "Transhumanism." In *New Bottles for New Wine: Essays*. London: Chatto & Windus, 1957.

Kass, Leon R. "Ageless Bodies, Happy Souls: Biotechnology and the Pursuit of Perfection." *The New Atlantis* (2003): 9–28.

Lossky, Vladimir. *In the Image and Likeness of God*, edited and translated by John H. Erikson and Thomas E. Bird. Crestwood, NY: St. Vladimir's Seminary Press, 1974.

Mehlman, Maxwell J. *The Price of Perfection: Individualism and Society in the Era of Biomedical Enhancement*. Baltimore: Johns Hopkins University Press, 2009.

Savulescu, Julian, and Anders Sandberg. "Neuroenhancement of Love and Marriage: The Chemicals Between Us." *Neuroethics* 1, no. 1 (2008): 31–44. www.springerlink.com/content/lp106323642w7062/fulltext.pdf.

Schneider, Susan. *Future Minds: Transhumanism, Cognitive Enhancement, and the Nature of Persons*. Center for Cognitive Neuroscience, 2008. http://ieet.org/archive/schneider01.pdf.

Chapter Two

Contextualizing a Christian Perspective on Transcendence and Human Enhancement

Francis Bacon, N. F. Fedorov, and Pierre Teilhard de Chardin

MICHAEL S. BURDETT

Transhumanism is the contemporary movement that advocates the use of technologies—biotechnology or information technology—to transcend what it means to be human. Its dependence upon cutting-edge technologies might make it seem to be a fairly recent phenomenon. Today's transhumanism has its antecedents, however, and its engagement with Christianity is not something that has only begun in the past decade. Although it is true that some Christian theologians have raised warnings about technology, it is equally true that other Christian intellectuals have promoted the use of technology, sometimes with a sense of urgency that rivals that of the transhumanists. Indeed, there is a strong tradition that does not see Christianity as at odds with human enhancement through technological means.

In this chapter I summarize the thought of three Christian thinkers who have advocated human enhancement through the avowal of technological and scientific means. First I turn to Francis Bacon, the English philosopher and political leader whose writings four hundred years ago profoundly shaped the rise of scientific culture. The next is N. F. Fedorov, whose work late in the nineteenth century was influential in his own time and is being rediscovered today. Finally I turn to the French paleontologist and Jesuit scholar Pierre Teilhard de Chardin, whose writings about the convergence of technology and theology were largely banned in his own lifetime but have become widely influential in recent decades, precisely because he was able to foresee some of the technological transformations that have occurred since his death in 1955. In their own way these thinkers regard technology as an important movement in Christian history itself—they advocate technological, human enhancement on Christian theological grounds.

Although Bacon, Fedorov, and Teilhard de Chardin are among the most important precursors of contemporary transhumanism to look favorably on transhumanism, others have made important contributions as well. For example, Freeman Dyson and Frank Tipler in the twentieth century come to mind, and perhaps one might even go as far back as Athanasius or Irenaeus and much of the Orthodox Christian tradition because of its avowal of divinization or *theosis*. The focus here, however, is on Bacon, Fedorov, and Teilhard de Chardin because these three represent, across some 350 years, major strides in bringing together contemporary transhumanism, with its emphasis on modern technology, and Christian practice and theology. Modern technology is a key component in their avowal of transhumanism, and their engagement with Christianity is not superficial but absolutely central to their advocacy of transhumanism.

Francis Bacon

Sir Francis Bacon (1561–1626) is a pivotal figure in both English political history and in philosophy and science. He has often been called the father of modernity and of contemporary science.[1] He wrote on a wide variety of topics spanning a number of academic disciplines. His most important work for our consideration is the *Instauratio Magna*, a work organized in six parts: *The Division of Sciences*, *The Novum Organon*, *The Phenomenon of the Universe*, *The Ladder of the Intellect*, *The Forerunners*, and *The New Philosophy*.[2] The term itself, *Instauratio Magna*, reveals how the work relates to transhumanism. This term was not in common use at the time and, in this way, points to the very specific way Bacon used it.[3] The term *instauration* is taken from the Vulgate and alludes to the restoration of Solomon's Temple.[4] So, whereas "establish" and "restore" might adequately translate the word *instauratio*, one must also recognize that for Bacon, the term carries a very particular connotation charged with symbolic values and religious undertones. What is being restored are human faculties that have been lost in the Fall. As Bacon states: "Both things can be repaired even in this life to some extent, the former by religion and faith, the latter by the arts and sciences. For the Curse did not make the creation an utter and irrevocable outlaw. In virtue of the sentence 'In the sweat of thy face shalt thou eat bread,' man, by manifold labours (and not by disputations, certainly, or by useless magical ceremonies), compels the creation, in time and in part, to provide him with bread, that is to serve the purposes of human life."[5]

Bacon's *Instauratio Magna* is supposed to help humanity limit the effects of its unredeemed state. The Fall brought with it alienation from God and a marred relationship with creation. Bacon held that the rift between God and humanity could only be remedied through supernatural and ecclesial means. Bridging the chasm separating humanity from Creation, however, was within the power of humanity. As Harrison claims, "In essence, this is how we are to understand Bacon's account of the two distinct ways in which there might be a restoration of what was lost at the Fall. While the loss of *innocence* could be restored only by grace, human *dominion*, made possible by Adamic knowledge, was not a supernatural gift but a natural capacity."[6] The *Instauratio Magna* is the formula Bacon proposes to restore the original human sovereignty over nature, which is evident in the book of Genesis. Regaining sovereignty over nature is central to Bacon's task, as is attested by Bacon's first usage of the term in an unpublished essay titled "Time's Masculine Birth, or the Great Instauration of Human Dominion over the Universe."[7]

Arguably, Bacon's most important work in the *Instauratio Magna* is the *Novum Organon*, or new instrument. In this text Bacon speaks of the specific ways in which humanity's fall from grace limits the reliability of what human beings can actually know about the world. Bacon refers to these imperfections or illusions as the idols. The first is the idol of the tribe. This idol describes the error that is inherent in perception itself and the limited and fallible nature of the human senses in general. The second idol is the idol of the cave. This idol refers to personal prejudice. People have a tendency to project onto the world what they think they ought to see instead of what is actually present. The third idol is the idol of the marketplace. This idol is best characterized and manifested in our common use of language. Language will sometimes fail to discriminate between distinctive phenomena. This could be due to the lack of the proper word, or the word could imply something that is not intended. Either way, the failure of language is a hindrance to perception and understanding. The final idol is that of the theater. This idol speaks of a failure in the actual system of belief itself. Idols of the theater "are the misleading consequences for human knowledge of the systems of philosophy and rules of demonstration (reliable proof) currently in place."[8]

The *Novum Organon* was precisely the new method that limits these idols. It was a qualitative and organized approach to the acquisition of reliable knowledge about the natural world, one that relied upon induction rather than tradition. This method began with an exhaustive formulation of lists of natural as well as experimental histories. The second step involved the organization of these histories into distinct tables so that one could gain access to them quickly and cross-reference with great ease. Once the tables were collimated and relationships between them were noted, certain phenomena could be induced. After a cycle of going through the tables, a claim could be made about the items in the table. From this first definition, a refining process of countless other experiments would make the tables even more specific and eventually lead to a more solid axiom that might look like our contemporary understanding of natural laws. It was through this method that reliable knowledge about nature was to be obtained, thereby limiting the effects of the idols and of the Fall.

Bacon's *Instauratio Magna* centers on this new method, which he believed would bring a golden age to humanity. The knowledge gained through this new method and its limiting of the effects of the Fall, however, were not its only benefits, according to him. He also wanted the information to be used in the construction of new technologies, which manifested the redeemed relationship between human beings and nature, repositioning humanity in its rightful location of dominion over nature.[9] The frontispiece of the *Instauratio Magna*, seen in figure 1, illustrates the anthropological significance Bacon attributed to his work. The image carries great symbolic significance. The two Pillars of Hercules represent the boundary between the known and unknown in the ancient world. The ship depicted represents two things related to the known and the unknown. The more literal interpretation suggests that Bacon was alluding to the great naval explorations of the fifteenth century. In this way, it represented human geographical advancement into the unknown. More important, however, is its natural and philosophical significance. The columns did not just represent the distinction between the known and the unknown; they also signified "the concept of the ancient cosmos in which man had a definite place in the order of things. Knowledge in this conception depended on discovery of the boundaries of man's nature so that he did not fall into a tragic life of wanton and animalic behaviour of sin or of sinful pride that caused him to overstep his boundaries and come into conflict with the gods."[10] What Bacon is alluding to in this image is an absolute transformation of humanity from a species confined by ancient myth to one that broaches upon the divine. For him humanity stood on the brink of a new epoch. The new method offered a way to regain our rightful place in the cosmos and to enjoy a more complete life in relation to both the world and God.

Bacon's other highly popularized text, *The New Atlantis*, seems to be related to this image as well. *The New Atlantis* begins with a ship blown off course into unknown waters. If the anthropological symbolism is carried through to this new text, then the new society represents what humanity would look like if it recovered some of its abilities lost in the Fall. Indeed, Bacon's utopia, written late in his life, projects what the world would be like if it followed Bacon's program.

The final part of *The New Atlantis*, which centers on Salomon's House, is the most important for our purposes. The society of Salomon's House is founded upon "the knowledge of Causes and secret motions of things; and the enlarging of the bounds of Human Empire, to the effecting of all

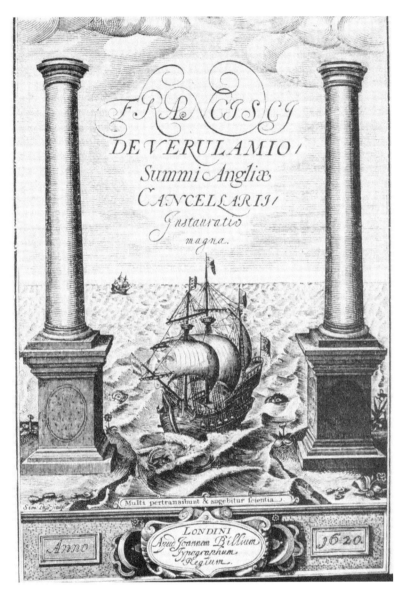

Figure 1. The frontispiece to Francis Bacon's 1620 *Instauratio Magna* showing a ship sailing between the metaphorical Pillars of Hercules at the Strait of Gibraltar from the classical world of the Mediterranean into the unexplored Atlantic. Image courtesy of History of Science Collections, University of Oklahoma libraries.

things possible."[11] It is a kind of priesthood that has unencumbered access to the book of Creation. It seeks to uncover the hidden natural laws so that humanity might benefit from the knowledge. For example, the sailors that stumble upon this utopian community learn that this society has massive subterranean halls, which are used for refrigeration and research on the production of new metals that can be employed for curing diseases and prolonging life.[12] The society of Salomon's House seems to be a mixture of scientific researchers and a religious or monastic order. Certain hermits live in these research caves and maintain a daily rite of prayer and observe other religious practices.[13] They also tend to wells and fountains that are used for medical purposes.[14] In this utopia the Baconian method, which emphasizes religion as well as science and technology, is at the very heart of the community.

Bacon founds his utopian vision upon more than just religious and scientific principles. The members of Salomon's House are religious scientists, but they are also skilled artisans who develop technical invention for the betterment of humanity. The society of Salomon's House does more than experiment for the knowledge of scientific laws; it has "engine-houses, where are prepared engines and instruments for all sorts of motion."[15] These houses contain all things mechanical, whether they are instruments of war or intricate clocks. These learned men are also well versed in mechanical arts and are skilled producers of paper, linen, and silk. In fact, the subdivision of labor in Salomon's House includes a group called the Benefactors whose sole purpose is to draw out of experimentation things for the practical use of the society.[16]

It is evident that religion, science, and technology are all important to Bacon's work. They all work together to raise the human species back to its rightful position as the lord over creation. Lewis Mumford comments on the significance of Bacon's contribution to the broad history of modern utopianism, beginning with Sir Thomas More (1478–1535):

> Though a whole literature of utopias soon followed in the wake of More's picture of an ideal commonwealth, it is significant that the only one whose direct effects can be traced was the mere fragment of a utopia left behind by Francis Bacon: for it was his *The New Atlantis* that first canvassed the possibility of a joint series of operations that would combine a new system of scientific investigation with a new technology. At a moment when the bitter struggle within Christianity between contentious doctrines and sects had come to a stalemate, the machine itself seemed to offer an alternative way of reaching Heaven. The promise of material abundance on earth, through exploration, organized conquest, and invention, offered a common objective to all classes.[17]

Through the employment of Baconian science and the technologies created from this method, human beings would no longer live at the mercy of nature but could rise to their proper place over it.

Nicolai Fedorovich Fedorov

Despite being little known in the West today, N. F. Fedorov (1828–1903) had many notable admirers of his work during his own lifetime, and his notoriety has only been increasing since the collapse of the Soviet Union. For instance, Dostoyevsky, in reference to Fedorov, wrote to N. P. Peterson, "First, a question: who is the thinker whose ideas you have transmitted? If you can, please let me know his real name. I have become so interested in him. . . . Secondly, I must say that in essence I completely agree with his ideas. I read them as if they were my own."[18] Fedorov is also said to have inspired the scene at Ilyusha's grave in Dostoyevsky's *The Brothers Karamazov*. The scene seems to be influenced by the central component of Fedorov's philosophy—complete bodily resurrection, something both Russian thinkers agreed on.[19] Furthermore, Leo Tolstoy, although not agreeing with Fedorov's project entirely, deeply respected Fedorov's ideas and his devotion to Christian practice. Tolstoy states: "Do not be afraid, I do not share his views, but I do understand them to such an extent that I feel capable of defending them and of giving them preference over any other views. Most important of all is the fact that, thanks to his belief, he leads a pure Christian life. Whenever I speak of the need of carrying out in real life the teachings of Christ, he says, 'but this is obvious,' and I know that with him it is so."[20] Other many notable philosophers and theologians—including Nikolai Berdyaev, Vladimir Solovev, and Vladimir Lossky—have admired Fedorov's gifted and creative mind and have agreed that he is a central figure in Russian theological and philosophical history.

Fedorov's major work, *The Philosophy of the Common Task*, was written in response to the general discord that Fedorov found between people and nature. As he noted, "Indeed, people have done all possible evil to nature (depletion, destruction, predatory exploitation) and to each other (inventing most abominable arms and implements of mutual extermination)."[21] Specifically, he cited the unbrotherly attitude people had toward one another, manifested in wars or in working for profit at the expense of their fellow man, or in the general selfishness and individualism rampant during his time. It was the tension between fellow human beings that most troubled him.

The Philosophy of the Common Task is a treatise that responds to this unbrotherly attitude, especially between the learned and the unlearned. As

Fedorov notes, "The hateful division of the world and all calamities that result from this compel us, the unlearned—that is, those who place action (action in common, not in strife) above thought—to submit to the learned this memorandum concerned with lack of kinship feelings and the means of restoring them."[22] In this sense, he saw his work as radically different from other philosophical tracts in that it was to provide the impetus for action in the world. He complained that the lofty transcendental writings of German philosophy, especially those of Kant, did not improve the actual conditions of the world, for this philosophy could not break free from the thinking mind to genuine action in the world. Philosophy was too caught up in the world of the mind without any real practical application for the common people.[23] The major problem Fedorov diagnosed was that education was not being used for the improvement of humankind as a whole but only to serve a select few. This exacerbated the gap between classes of human beings.

Fedorov claimed that most of the problems that exist between humans are directly related to the struggle humanity has with its own primitive nature. Indeed, many of the philosophical and ideological underpinnings of Fedorov's *Philosophy of the Common Task* depend upon how humanity has become distinct from animals. This distinction is most evident in the human assumption of a vertical posture. Fedorov sees great significance in the act of walking upright. In this action, humanity literally moves away from the forces of nature on the ground, asserting the first real act of will. As he claims, "Creatures who face the earth, which is covered with vegetation and is inhabited by other creatures, have only one aim, namely, to devour vegetation or these other creatures. . . . On the other hand, the vertical posture of man is above all an expression of man's revulsion from this need to devour. Indeed, the vertical posture is man's endeavour to raise himself above the destructiveness which prevails in Nature."[24]

This first act of will also implies the beginning of selfhood for humanity. It is precisely in opposition to nature that human beings distinguish themselves, becoming subjects.[25] It is this cleavage from the animal kingdom, whereby the individual slowly distinguishes himself or herself as a person, that transforms the animal fear of death into its more robust and abstract equivalent in this now conscious person. Death is now seen as the destruction of personal identity and freedom from the forces of nature. It is not a biological death that is important for Fedorov's appraisal of primitive humanity, but the destruction of the individual's own self-creation in freedom from nature and a primitive past.

Fedorov then takes up this polarity inherent in the primitive human, this transcendence of humanity in opposition to the forces of nature, as the basis for his philosophical task. His main argument is that the discord that exists in the world can be alleviated through unification against the common enemy, death. As Berdyaev states, "For Nikolai Fedorov the one and the ultimate evil is death. Every evil derives from death and leads to death. The world-wide struggle against death is the problem confronting mankind."[26] In fact, Fedorov was so opposed to death that he would rarely sleep longer than a few hours at night because it reminded him of death.[27] Death is the ultimate enemy of humankind and "is not a quality which determines *what a human being is and must be*" (emphasis added).[28]

Unifying all humanity against the common enemy of death, as abstract as this sounds, has a very practical element. Fedorov claimed that as humanity has arisen from the natural world—indeed, it is even defined by this will to break free from nature—uniting humanity against death has come to mean regulating this blind force of nature. He sought to alleviate problems of warfare, not by avowing pacifism and disbanding standing armies as his compatriot Tolstoy did, but by advocating that resources and energy be redirected from war toward the scientific study of the Earth and regulating it for humanity's ends. Fedorov suggested that the great military weapons could be used to manipulate weather patterns to increase crop yields or to limit some natural disasters by setting off explosions in the atmosphere.[29] He was not unfounded in this assertion at the time. Scientific experiments were being conducted by the Americans to control weather, and even today both the Russians and Chinese have put significant funding into cloud seeding.[30] He also suggested that massive cables be placed around the Earth to manipulate its magnetic field and control the amount of solar radiation.[31] Additionally, he did not want to limit humanity's regulation of nature to just the planet Earth, but he also foresaw the need to transform the Earth from a piece of rock at the mercy of cosmic forces to one harnessed by humanity so that it might be a "terrestrial craft" from which humanity's exploration and management of the cosmos had no bounds.[32]

Fedorov's rejection of death as a necessary condition for humanity moved beyond just conquering the cosmos through human reason. More important for him was the absolute cessation of death for humanity and the material resurrection of all its ancestors. This imperative, although grounded in the desire for human unification, ultimately stems from his Christian faith. It is true that he insisted that humans should control nature for their own assertion of freedom and personhood, but this is always and everywhere a response based on the Christian message. Christianity is the religion of resurrection, and even the resurrection of ancestors is important for him.

Death and its overcoming in the resurrection lie at the center of the Christian narrative. What is distinctive about Fedorov's interpretation of the resurrection is that it is both a complete material and bodily resurrection and also a task meant to be enacted by humanity. The resurrection is not relegated to mere spiritual abstraction, nor does it lie in the hands of God alone. As Berdyaev states, "According to Fedorov's doctrine, the resurrection of the dead is achieved not only through action accomplished by Christ, the Redeemer and Saviour, and not only by the spiritual and moral efforts of mankind and the love of human beings for the deceased, but also by the scientific, technical, and physical activity of people. By the joint efforts of religion and science, of priest and learned technician, the dead and buried must experience their resurrection. Fedorov even speaks about the physico-chemical experiments of resurrecting the dead, which produces an almost frightening impression."[33]

Human action in resurrecting the ancestors stems from Fedorov's rejection of Monophysitic Christology and the sacred continuity between creation and God's life in the Trinity.[34] Monophysitic Christianity denies the human element in the Incarnation by asserting a single divine nature. This is insufficient for Fedorov because it makes the transformation of nature ultimately a divine action rather than one which humanity can contribute. Orthodox Christianity emphasizes the transformation of the Earth into the glorified creation God intends. Like so many other Eastern Christians, Fedorov took a distinctly materialistic approach to this transformation, but he also suggested science and technology as the means by which this should occur. He claimed that unique individual vibrations (similar to resonance frequency) exist for each person, even following death. These could be manipulated in such a way that they could be reunited with their "solid-state molecules on Earth."[35] He was clear, however, that resurrection was much more than just technological manipulation of matter but was to be rooted in the love that was modeled in the Trinity and that sought to conform this world to the life of God.[36]

Fedorov's entire project hinges upon the utilization of science and technology for the universal and material resurrection of all humanity. His philosophy is premised upon the rejection of death as a central aspect of the human condition. He has defined humanity precisely in distinction from other animals through the rejection of death. The human species is a transcending animal that must subdue the forces of blind nature for its own survival and identity. For Fedorov the essence of the Christian message and the commission of humanity is to practice this defiance toward nature through material resurrection and by controlling all natural forces.

Pierre Teilhard de Chardin

Pierre Teilhard de Chardin (1881–1955), the final figure under consideration, was a French Jesuit and trained paleontologist who became one of the first people to combine evolutionary theory with Christian theology. In his works on paleontology he takes seriously the force of technology. It is in reflecting upon the human future that he advocates the enhancement of humanity through technological means. To understand how technology functions in his thought, it is best to consider his eschatology. He gives three distinct features that will be important to the formation of the future to the eschaton.

First, Teilhard claims that social unification will continue to occur among diverse races and peoples. He claims that "nothing . . . can arrest the progress of social Man toward greater interdependence and cohesion."[37] This trend toward unification is a function of the limited space on our planet.[38] Humanity has flourished and spread around the globe like no other species. This inevitably leaves less space for people to exist. As the density of the population increases, how do human beings adapt? Teilhard suggests that historically when this has occurred, it has led to a restructuring of the species in greater organization. We see this taking place in cities around the world. Cities are forced to organize a great amount of resources—food, energy, infrastructure—in order for such a dense population to exist and persist in such a small area. This trend will only increase in the future, as the world becomes one unified society that has learned to adapt to a limited space.[39]

Second, the future will continue in its mechanization, a process that does not seem to be going away, but only speeding up. Technology is a major force in human development. For Teilhard, technology represents "the sum of processes combined reflectively in such a way as to preserve in men the state of consciousness which corresponds to our state of aggregation and conjunction."[40] In other words, as the human species has evolved from a more simple state, its utilization and creation of technology has allowed it to interact with its environment in a very flexible way. Whereas other species have relied upon their bodily advantage (e.g., claws, speed, exoskeleton) to escape predators, humanity had to rely upon complex behaviors rather than instincts. This allowed humanity not to be imprisoned in its own body but free to develop cognitively. Technology and consciousness are in a symbiotic relationship, which finds its most simplistic roots in the coherence of the mind and body itself. Technology represents the external counterpart which consciousness relies upon for its own propagation. Human consciousness not only creates these technologies but even relies upon them for its own evolution. Technology merely makes the relation between the mind and the external world more efficient and productive. For Teilhard claims, "What has really let loose the Machine in the world, and for good, is that it both facilitates and indefinitely multiplies our activities. Not only does it relieve us mechanically of a crushing weight of physical and mental labour, but by the miraculous enhancing of our senses, through the powers of enlargement, penetration and exact measurement, it constantly increases the scope and clarity of our perceptions. It fulfils the dream of all living creatures by satisfying our instinctive craving for *the maximum consciousness* with a minimum of effort!" (emphasis added).[41] It is clear for Teilhard that in using technology, conscious human beings are freed from the confines of mundane tasks to navigate the world.

Furthermore, not only does technology indirectly aid human development through reduced effort, but it can also be used to enhance humanity directly. Teilhard recognized this possibility and suggested that biologists would one day be able to manipulate human chromosomes, or that psychoanalysis might lead to the modification of basic human instincts and thought.[42] He states: "This power means that mankind holds in its hands the means of varying the complexity of the focus on which its whole future depends."[43] People thus could directly manipulate the complexity of their own bodies and have direct influence on their own transformation. This ability represents a major step in humanity's control over its own future, and by extension the future of the world.

Third, the final trend that will lead humanity into the future is a heightening of vision.[44] This heightened vision not only refers to the greater advancement in our technologies that reveal more phenomena but also to our general enhancement of the knowledge of the universe because of this increase in faculties. The compression of the human population leads to greater socialization, unification, and technologization, not only for the sake of survival but also for the increased freedom of respective individuals. As duties become more compartmentalized in society and trivial tasks are made obsolete, mental effort can be devoted elsewhere. This heightening of vision is exactly what Teilhard suggests that humanity does with its surplus psychic energy by researching more and developing technology.

All these tendencies lead Teilhard to assert that the world is in a state of convergence and unification, and thus is moving toward what he calls the Omega Point. Integrally related to this convergence toward the Omega Point is his understanding of what he calls personalization. Each individual grows and evolves, becoming more of an individual with greater consciousness. This greater consciousness leads to a more defined center in each person. What is most important to note is that this individual personalization is not divorced from the exterior environment in which the person grows.

These personal centers are not only centers for the individual human but also represent the greater centricity of the entire world and milieu in which personalization occurs. The personality created in human consciousness is merely the more complex form of atomization in the world more generally. In this way, not only are human individuals ontically distinct from their primordial counterparts, but they are also related in the general trend of personalization.[45]

This distinction is intensified by the formation and enrichment of the Noosphere. Teilhard understands the Noosphere as the collective mind of humanity as thought emerges and becomes increasingly unified. It is a way of looking at the phenomenon of communal thought, but from the planetary level. The cerebral element of the Noosphere not only refers to each individual mind within the Noosphere but even to the greater centricity that exists in the Noosphere as an entity in its own right, as a kind of planetary mind. As Teilhard states, "All our difficulties and repulsions as regards the opposition between the All and the Person would be dissipated if only we understood that, by structure, the Noosphere (and more generally the world) represent a whole that is not only closed but also centered."[46] Indeed, personalization is occurring to the Noosphere itself, a process that Teilhard calls Noogenesis. Every individual within the collectivity of the human race is increasing in his or her own personalization, while this very collectivity is converging toward its own person. This is where Teilhard's distinction between personality and individuality plays a key role. Personalization differentiates amid a total union, whereas individualization separates itself at the expense of the whole and leads to greater plurality. Individuality sacrifices the ultrapersonal element of humanity at large. For Teilhard, personalization is the proper way to the future as it cultivates the personal element of the Noosphere. Individuality, conversely, leads to separation, divergence, and ultimately death.

Teilhard asserts that the Noosphere is the most important strand in the progression of the universe and humanity to the end of history. It is the force of personalization in the Noosphere that is the foundation of his eschatology. As he states, "The only air which Reflection can breathe must, of vital necessity, be that of a psychically and physically convergent Universe. There must be some peak, some revelation, some vivifying transformation at the end of the journey."[47] As the Noosphere becomes more centered, it leads to the creation of a person. The *telos* of this convergence in the Noosphere points to a particular person, whom Teilhard refers to as the Ultra-Human or the Trans-Human. Everything immanent within the cosmos is funneling its energy toward a single point at the end of history. This Omega Point is reached through "the push" of evolutionary forces and "the pull," which rests on the attraction of the Omega Point today in the affinity that people have for each other in mutual love.

The end of history lies where humanity converges into the completed person of the cosmic Christ. This occurs through an escape from the cosmos and separation of the material world at its termination of history. As Noogenesis, the development of the Noosphere, reaches its maturity, the material world is jettisoned. This is the final act before the Omega Point is reached and the Ultra-Human is drawn up into the supernatural Christ. This final union speaks to the ontological distinction and priority that Teilhard sees between the supernatural and the natural. Naturalistic evolution, though leading to the final consummation with the divine, is not itself the final movement into the divine. It is the necessary precondition for its final unity with God. As Teilhard states, "By structural necessity, the two points inevitably coincide—in this sense, that the fulfilment of hominisation by ultra-reflection is seen to be a necessary pre-condition of its 'divinisation.'"[48] The final development of the Ultra-Human is the penultimate act at the eschaton, when God alone brings humanity to glory and divinization.

It is through the utilization of technology among other trends associated with humanity that the human species is progressing toward a particular point of convergence in history. Teilhard advocates that these trends should be bolstered and encouraged. Specifically, he is a firm supporter of not only the socially unifying effects of technology but also even their use for human biological enhancement. He affirms this on theological grounds: When one enhances humanity, it is a further step in the drive toward the consummation of humanity and the universal Christ.

Conclusion

It is apparent that there is a tradition within Christian history that does not see the enhancement of humanity through technological means as a particular problem. As we have seen, Bacon advises that his new science would mitigate the effects of the Fall and enhance humanity's dominion over the world. Fedorov claims that death is the ultimate enemy of humanity and that its limitation through technological resurrection should be the aim of humanity and the Christian. Teilhard de Chardin encourages the use of technology to enhance humanity, because he believes that each biological step is advancing toward the cosmic Christ. These three figures represent a strand in Christendom extending from the sixteenth to twentieth centuries that recognized the growing possibilities that spring from technology and its ability to transform humanity. All three have incorporated this affirmation of technology into their Christian vision and even advocated the usage of technology to enhance humanity on Christian grounds. When considering the contemporary issues of bio-enhancement and technological transcendence from a Christian perspective, it is instructive to remember that the Christian tradition is marked with a multiplicity of positions and that a simple reactionary stance is not the only strand within Christian history.

Notes

1. For biographical information and his relation to modernity, see Peltonen, "Bacon"; and Whitney, *Francis Bacon*.

2. Peltonen, "Introduction," 15.

3. Whitney, "Francis Bacon's *Instauratio*," 371.

4. Ibid.

5. Bacon, *New Organon*, 221.

6. Harrison, *Fall of Man*, 158.

7. Whitney, "Francis Bacon's *Instauratio*," 371.

8. Jardine, "Introduction," xix–xx.

9. See Nanni, "Technical Knowledge."

10. McKnight, *Science, Pseudo-Science, and Utopianism*, 111.

11. Bacon, *Advancement of Learning*, 239.

12. Ibid.

13. Ibid., 247.

14. Ibid., 240.

15. Ibid., 244.

16. Ibid., 246.

17. Mumford, *Myth of the Machine*, 283.

18. Dostoyevsky, "Appendix I," 227.

19. Koutaissoff, "Introduction," 15.

20. For a partial translation of Tolstoy's letter to A. I. Alexeev, see Lukashevich, *N. F. Fedorov*, 22.

21. Fedorov, *What Was Man Created For?* 34.

22. Ibid., 39.

23. Ibid., 46–51.

24. See Lukashevich, *N. F. Fedorov*, 47, for a translation of Nikolai Fedorovich Fedorov, *Filosofiia Obshchago Dela* (Moscow, 1913), vol. 2, 264, 265.

25. Lukashevich, *N. F. Fedorov*, 47–48.

26. Berdyaev, "N. F. Fedorov," 125.

27. Lukashevich, *N. F. Fedorov*, 18.

28. Fedorov, *What Was Man Created For?* 99.

29. Ibid., 148–50.

30. For the details of the American scientific experiments to which Fedorov refers, see ibid., 144–58; and Koutaissoff, "Introduction," 27–28. On Russia and China's attempts to cloud seed, see Engber, "Can the Russians Control Weather?"; and Aiyar, "Ready, Aim."

31. Fedorov, *What Was Man Created For?* 95.

32. Ibid., 97.

33. Berdyaev, "Fedorov," 128.

34. Ibid., 126.

35. Fedorov, *What Was Man Created For?* 193.

36. Ibid., 193–94; Berdyaev, "Fedorov," 127.

37. Teilhard de Chardin, *Future of Man*, 226.

38. Ibid.

39. See also Teilhard de Chardin, *Activation of Energy*, 341–46.

40. Ibid., 159.

41. Teilhard de Chardin, *Future of Man*, 227.

42. Teilhard de Chardin, *Activation of Energy*, 160.

43. Ibid.

44. Teilhard de Chardin, *Future of Man*, 227–28.

45. See esp. Teilhard de Chardin, *Human Energy*, 53–60.

46. Teilhard de Chardin, *Phenomenon of Man*, 285.

47. Teilhard de Chardin, *Future of Man*, 278.

48. Teilhard de Chardin, *Toward the Future*, 191.

References

Aiyar, Pallavi. "Ready, Aim, Fire and Rain." *Asia Times*, July 13, 2007.

Bacon, Francis. *The Advancement of Learning and the New Atlantis*. Oxford: Oxford University Press, 1974.

———. *The New Organon*, edited by Lisa Jardine and Michael Silverthorne. Cambridge: Cambridge University Press, 2000.

Berdyaev, Nicholas. "N. F. Fedorov." *Russian Review* 9, no. 2 (1950): 124–30.

Dostoyevsky, Fyodor. "Appendix I." In *What Was Man Created For? The Philosophy of the Common Task: Selected Works*, 227–29. London: Honeyglen, 1990.

Engber, Daniel. "Can the Russians Control Weather? How Cloud Seeding Works." *Slate*, May 11, 2005.

Fedorov, Nikolai Fedorovich. *Filosofiia Obshchago Dela*, vol. 2. Moscow, 1913.

———. *What Was Man Created For? The Philosophy of the Common Task: Selected Works*, translated by Elisabeth Koutaissoff and Marilyn Minto. London: Honeyglen, 1990.

Harrison, Peter. *The Fall of Man and the Foundations of Science*. Cambridge: Cambridge University Press, 2007.

Jardine, Lisa. "Introduction." In *The New Organon*, edited by Lisa Jardine and Michael Silverthorne. Cambridge: Cambridge University Press, 2000.

Koutaissoff, Elisabeth. "Introduction." In *What Was Man Created For? The Philosophy of the Common Task: Selected Works*. London: Honeyglen, 1990.

Lukashevich, Stephen. *N. F. Fedorov (1828–1903): A Study of Russian Eupsychian and Utopian Thought*. Newark: University of Delaware Press, 1977.

McKnight, Stephen A., ed. *Science, Pseudo-Science, and Utopianism in Early Modern Thought*. Columbia: University of Missouri Press, 1992.

Mumford, Lewis. *The Myth of the Machine*. London: Secker & Warburg, 1967.

Nanni, Romano. "Technical Knowledge and the Advancement of Learning: Some Questions about 'Perfectability' and 'Invention.'" In *Philosophies of Technology: Francis Bacon and His Contemporaries*, edited by Claus Zittel. Leiden: Brill, 2008.

Peltonen, Markku. "Bacon, Francis, Viscount St Alban (1561–1626)." In *Oxford Dictionary of National Biography*, edited by H. C. G. Matthew and Brian Harrison. Oxford: Oxford University Press, 2004.

———. "Introduction." In *The Cambridge Companion to Francis Bacon*, edited by Markku Peltonen. Cambridge: Cambridge University Press, 1996.

Teilhard de Chardin, Pierre. *Activation of Energy*, translated by René Hague. London: Collins, 1970.

———. *The Future of Man*, translated by Norman Denny. New York: Doubleday Image Books, 2004.

———. *Human Energy*, translated by J. M. Cohen. London: Collins, 1969.

———. *The Phenomenon of Man*, translated by Bernard Wall. London: Fontana, 1965.

———. *Toward the Future*, translated by René Hague. London: Collins, 1975.

Whitney, Charles. *Francis Bacon and Modernity*. New Haven, CT: Yale University Press, 1986.

———. "Francis Bacon's *Instauratio*: Dominion of and over Humanity." *Journal of the History of Ideas* 50, no. 3 (1989): 371–90.

Chapter Three

Transformation and the End of Enhancement

Insights from Pierre Teilhard de Chardin

DAVID GRUMETT

F ew theologians have offered more suggestive openings for a constructive dialogue with transhumanism than the French Jesuit Pierre Teilhard de Chardin. Because he was also a paleontologist, he sensed deeply the
dynamic of evolutionary development that has shaped the world from its
origins, and he recognized that human beings have become agents of their
own evolution. Having been born in 1881, he was prophetic in his realization
that technology and human intelligence were beginning to combine to produce a potent new transformative force in biological, mental, and spiritual
life.

The lack of engagement by transhumanists with Teilhard is surprising. In
his short history of the movement, Nick Bostrom gives him a passing mention but no substantive assessment, attributing to him a vague mysticism of
encroaching global consciousness.[1] But Teilhard presents a far more nuanced
vision than this, especially in his later writings dating from about 1940 until
his death in 1955. It is on these later texts that this chapter focuses.

The transhumanists' neglect of Teilhard has recently been redressed by
the philosopher Eric Steinhart, who in an excellent article developing a computational interpretation of Teilhard's oeuvre sees a high degree of coinci-
dence between his thought and that of present-day transhumanism, even
suggesting that Teilhard points the way to a "Christian transhumanism."[2]
Nevertheless, it needs to be stated clearly that Teilhard would not accept
all the transhumanists' assumptions and values, and could not himself be
described as a "transhumanist" without careful qualification. This makes
him an ideal partner for a critical but constructive conversation with the
transhumanists.

I cannot in this chapter address the full breadth of transhumanist thought,
and thus for reasons of space I generalize, mainly making direct compari-
sons with the work of two of its leading exponents, Ray Kurzweil and Nick
Bostrom. This enables me to evaluate some of the theological and ethical

notions underlying transhumanism as exemplified by these exponents. It also allows me to identify points of convergence and divergence with Christian theology as expressed in the oeuvre of Teilhard. I first examine the common ground that is obviously shared by Teilhard and the transhumanists, before assessing the metaphysical, ethical, and theological constraints that, he believed, placed boundaries around human technological transformations of the world and of humanity itself. I then appraise some specific transhumanist ends, and offer concluding comments comparing these with classic Christian conceptions of transcendence.

Teilhard and Transhumanism

As already noted, Teilhard could easily be presented as a prototypical transhumanist. Indeed, in an essay first published in 1951 he employs similar terminology, referring in his closing sentence to "some sort of trans-humanity at the ultimate heart of things."[3] Moreover, it is likely that he influenced the terminology of Julian Huxley, who is often credited with coining the term "transhuman" in a short chapter published six years later.[4] The two were close friends and collaborated during the period when Huxley was developing his evolutionary synthesis, despite their opposing views on whether evolution had a direction.[5]

Nonetheless, the degree of convergence should not be overstated at this opening stage of the discussion, not least to maintain a constructive critical distance between Christian theology and transhumanism. In opening, I therefore propose that Teilhard and the transhumanists are limited to seven points of convergence. First, they agree that biological evolution exhibits direction and purpose. Teilhard describes this as a "cosmic slide from the simple to the complex."[6] Kurzweil's epochal theory also posits evolutionary intelligence, design, and order.[7] Second, humans stand at the end point of biological evolution, and no nonhuman species will evolve from humans.[8] There will be many future advances in human life, but these will not be impelled by classic biological mechanisms. Rather, they will be due to technological innovation and shifts in human consciousness. As Kurzweil emphatically puts it, human centrality will continue "until the entire universe is at our fingertips."[9]

Third, Teilhard and transhumanists agree that human history exhibits direction and purpose. This is primarily the result of technological development and the associated expansion and intensification of reflection. Teilhard usually describes the latter as an expansion in consciousness, whereas Bostrom expresses a similar vision of the accumulation of instrumentally useful information.[10] Fourth, knowledge, intelligence, and reflection are increasingly powerful shapers of identity and development. When evolution was biological, intelligence functioned primarily as a survival mechanism. But intelligence is becoming far more important in human life, to the extent that it will be the chief factor governing further human development.[11] This is especially apparent in Kurzweil's fifth and sixth epochs of evolution.[12]

Fifth, Teilhard and the transhumanists agree that centers of consciousness are multiplying and converging as humanity acquires ever greater collective reflective capacity.[13] Teilhard coined the term "Noosphere" to describe a conscious network encircling the Earth. Kurzweil pictures the World Wide Web as "information swirl[ing] around the globe oblivious to borders of any kind."[14] Sixth, they agree that new phases in human life have been heralded by points of exponential transition. Teilhard describes the earliest human life as the result of a "breakthrough of reflection" that suddenly transformed the nature of sentience and engendered thought; the birth of the Noosphere marks an analogous radical shift in consciousness.[15] In his epochal theory, Kurzweil posits a succession of paradigm shifts and presents the "Singularity" as a time of technological change of rapid pace and deep impact.[16] And finally, they agree that human life does not consist in a fixed, immutable essence of humanity. Rather, human life is in a process of ongoing transformation, and humanity's freedom to determine its own evolutionary future is increasing.[17] Teilhard would accept Bostrom's assessment of human nature as a work in progress.[18] This does not mean that humans have been created deficiently, but simply that creation is continuing.

Teilhard thus accepts the broad transhumanist consensus that evolution is directional, in both its prehuman and human phases, and that human life marks its end point. He recognizes the rapidly increasing potency of reflection in shaping the world through human ingenuity and collective human consciousness. He identifies periods of exponential change in human life and believes that humanity is currently passing through such a period, as part of a wider movement of ongoing transformation.

The Goals of Transformation

What are the goals of human transformation? These can be seen from two perspectives: the goals of individual humans, and the goals of evolution itself. In this section, I reflect on overarching evolutionary goals, and I reserve consideration of concrete ethical ends for the subsequent section.

Discerning the broad goals of evolution involves paying attention to the design and patterning of the world's development. Teilhard believes that these reveal several metaphysical principles. Human life is increasingly compressed and socialized on a scale that is global, bounded by geographical and mental "curvatures" beyond which it cannot advance. The first curvature is due to the simple fact of inhabiting a planet of finite surface area. The second arises from the interconnections created by rationality and the technological networks that it generates.[19] These globalized networks are now as inescapable as the planet itself. A major reality of future human life will be the concentration of more people, ideas, and expectations on the planet's surface. Teilhard regards human colonization of other planets or solar systems as unlikely due to insurmountable technical challenges as well as the absence on Earth of colonists from any other planet.[20]

Internal impulsion is just as significant to human life as external limitation. Because he is influenced at this point by the vitalism of Henri Bergson, Teilhard sees a "will to subsist and grow greater" as fundamental to human existence.[21] His clear emphasis on the role of personal agents in initiating or at least mediating new intellectual and technological development provides an important corrective to narratives of inexorable, triumphant cosmic advance into which individual humans are involuntarily swept. The imagination and spontaneity on which invention depends emerge from real reflective acts originating in real human communities.

Human life is continually acquiring greater complexity. Anticipating systems theory, Teilhard describes a twofold process of radiation and attraction whereby systems exponentially develop more interconnections, and he applies this model both to human mental development and external human systems such as political units and the emerging world order. In the individual human mind—insofar as the mind can still be regarded as separable from the larger information networks in which it participates—the result is more profound thought patterns, whereas in the wider world such multiplication allows enhanced communication and reflection globally. Teilhard observes: "We can see connexions of all sorts continually—and in geometric progression—multiplying and intensifying between each human individual and all the others on the surface of the globe."[22] Each element thus becomes interlinked with every other one, and in this sense "rapidly co-extensive with the whole surface of the globe."[23]

Humans are conscious, and a global consciousness is produced by the network of links and interactions between them. Nevertheless, to interpret either human or global life solely as a network is to fail to identify the element of contingency that makes human and earthly life unique. This inherent unpredictability is a consequence of the irreducibly personal dimension of both God and human life. In consequence, humans are called to promote true reflectivity and the concrete activities from which personality emerges, such as imagination, artistic expression, creativity, prayer, and vision.[24] Human and theological goods such as these cannot be interpreted merely as functions of a universal connectivity. They are manifestations of the mental and spiritual life of specific humans, and they need to be recognized and nurtured as such. It is clear even in the present day that some complex systems—whether people, physical spaces, or organizations—exhibit far greater reflectivity than others, such as by generous acts of hospitality or through inspiring people who interact with them. Although it might well be possible to accommodate such values within the framework of information theory, any description of them solely in these terms will fail to account for their intrinsic worth, especially in generating new ethical and spiritual goods.

Evolution will develop progressively more spiritualized forms. Yet future human existence, although spiritual, will not be nonmaterial. Teilhard envisions not a "breakaway from matter" but a "passing through and emerging from matter," and he thus frequently warns against models of humanity that fail to recognize its continued dependence on matter.[25] As a result of his paleontological work, he realized that, in all phases of evolution, spiritual growth is manifested materially. More important, however, the essential nature of humankind as comprising both matter and spirit is a theological doctrine revealed in the Incarnation, whereby Jesus Christ was sent by the Father as his spiritual principle into the world to assume a fully human, material body.

In contrast to this strongly incarnational view of the soul as both material and spiritual, the transhumanists tend to regard the soul in excessively abstract spiritual terms. In so doing, they unwittingly follow a strand of Christian reflection originating in the need perceived by Thomas Aquinas and other scholastic theologians from the thirteenth century onward that the soul be separable from the body. This was in order that the graced soul would be able to enter the state of purgatory, in which it would be purified of its venial sins in order to grow in holiness and thus be ready to enter Heaven. This tradition is in contrast with Paul's insistence in 1 Corinthians 15:35–57 that the resurrected spiritual body, though not "physical," is still a "body" and not a pattern of information or a disembodied mind. The perishable, mortal body *puts on* imperishability and immortality, rather than divesting itself of materiality.

Future evolution can be understood as an analogical repetition of past evolutionary developments. Teilhard uses the image of the "breakthrough of reflection" at the birth of humanity as a model for the growth of global reflectivity in the Western world of the mid–twentieth century.[26] Although the latter idea is in many ways identifiable with Kurzweil's Singularity concept, Teilhard understands the Singularity not as an event entirely unlike anything preceding. Rather, he sees present-day shifts in the nature of consciousness as repetitions in concentrated form of the evolutionary shift that occurred with the original emergence of reflection in *Homo sapiens*, which constituted the birth of humankind. Furthermore, whereas Kurzweil sees the Singularity as unique, for Teilhard it cannot be the ultimate end of human transformation. I return to this key contested point below.

The Ethical Ends of Humanity

In transhumanist discourse, the moral ends that humans should pursue are set within a general metaphysics with many similarities to those just described above. This grounding of ethics in metaphysics—that is, in the analysis of fundamental principles such as being, knowing, identity, and change—marks a refreshing and important break with the tendency in recent decades to derive ethical norms from principles abstracted from any scientific or other empirical analysis of the world. Yet no such analysis is value neutral, least of all the transhumanist analysis with its high valuation of purpose and spiritual connectedness. Moreover, moral reasoning also bears a necessary circularity, because it is necessarily founded on observation and reasoning.[27] Morals can no more be considered in separation from metaphysics than metaphysics can be detached from morals. I now begin to develop a more critical assessment of transhumanism by comparing and contrasting the more concrete ethical ends implicit in transhumanist and Teilhardian metaphysics.

Fundamental to the transhumanist worldview is the accelerating growth of intelligence and reflection. As already intimated, however, this large-scale growth cannot be abstracted from the intelligent, reflective lives of real human beings. On the contrary, reflection by such human beings is essential given the vastly expanded power of their activities, when technologically harnessed, for either good or ill. Indeed, Bostrom (writing with Milan Ćirković) admits in the introduction to a collection surveying possible future apocalypses that "the most likely global catastrophic risks all seem to arise from human activities, especially industrial civilization and advanced technologies."[28] Various contributors refer to activities and capacities that have classically been regarded as elements of the ethical life such as education, training, imagination, conceptualization, and attentiveness. Nevertheless, no coherent ethical response to the various possible catastrophes under consideration is developed. This seems strange, given that Bostrom's statement is important and, for the theologian or ethicist, obvious. Ethics seems, in contrast, to be regarded as at best an epiphenomenon of material, technical reality and pragmatic responses to it.

The central role of ethical human agents in promoting an intelligent, reflective world is so great that Teilhard rightly sees them as cocreators with

God. In view of the modern realization that the world is continually evolving and changing, it would be wrong to regard creation as a once-for-all completed divine act. Rather, it is an ongoing reality. The notion of cocreation is
not, of course, incompatible with the idea that a single act of divine creation
brought the world into being. On the contrary, the original creative event
caused by God's free will marks the beginning of a creative process. Teilhard states: "There is not one moment when God creates, and one moment
when the secondary causes develop. There is always only *one* creative action
(identical with conservation) which continually raises creatures towards
fuller-being, *by means of* their secondary activity and their earlier advances.
Understood in this way, creation is not a period intrusion of the First Cause:
It is an act co-extensive with the whole duration of the universe."[29]

Human participation in divine creative activity is thus linked with the
notion that creation is cumulative. As the above quotation makes clear, however, creation does not cease to be a single divine action. Nevertheless, from
a temporal perspective, creation is an action dispersed through space and
time.

Teilhard's vision of technology contributing to the realization of God's
purpose for the world does not imply naive approval of every technical
innovation or process. Instead, it helps to establish a normative standard
against which these can and should be judged, informed by the theological metaphysics previously described. Technical projects that fail to concord
with God's will for the world cannot be regarded as cooperating with that
will. In particular, the function of humans as cocreators with God imposes
limits on human innovation. This is articulated with particular clarity in a
discussion of the "moral ordering of invention." Teilhard defines invention
broadly, not simply as scientific discovery but as "everything in human activity which in one way or another contributes to the organico-social construction of the Noosphere and the development within it of new powers for
the arrangement of Matter."[30] This construction is necessarily guided by
the metaphysics described in the previous section, and it is governed by two
ethical principles: respect for the things produced, and for the personality of
the people producing them.

Nevertheless, given the expanding gulf between technical and moral
progress in the modern world, both these principles are frequently disre-
garded. Ethical principles are still too often seen, Teilhard argues, as a means
of imposing external restrictions on future development. In fact he shows
that ethics is, in the present day, nothing less than a condition for the survival
of the human race—not in the sense of preventing further changes by preserving the technological status quo but as essential to inspiring and directing future development. He states that "evolution, in *rebounding* reflectively

upon itself, acquires *morality* for the purpose of its further advance."[31] The reflective arrangement this generates is "charged with internal obligations which curb and direct it." In other words, human technical endeavor needs ethics. Any technological enterprise should nevertheless have clear spiritual ends in sight: Progress does not consist in simply any technological novelty or expansion of humans' power over their material or social environment. Rather, progress is the enlargement of reflective and moral capacity.

The general notion that evolution exhibits wisdom that humans should recognize and with which they should, in their scientific endeavor, cooperate is by no means absent from transhumanist discussion. Moreover, exponents acknowledge the specific need to promote social as well as individual well-being.[32] Yet concrete proposals typically privilege enhancements of a physical variety, such as the engineering of stronger skeletons and teeth, optimizing the proportion of red blood cells in the human body, or disevolving the appendix.[33] Teilhard himself also identifies the central importance of addressing aspects of humankind's material condition, such as combating mass infections, generating sufficient energy to meet future needs, and feeding the world's population by converting carbon, nitrogen, and other simple elements directly into food.[34] But he generally places greater value on measures that will increase human socialization, such as improvements in global communications and reflective capacity.[35] He would therefore be sympathetic to many practical aspects of Kurzweil's vision of future evolutionary development, but with significant reservations about the metaphysical assumptions framing it. In the final section, I consider these deeper assumptions.

Death, Transcendence, and Immortality

Teilhard describes the growth of complex systems of collective self-consciousness (co-reflection) as "ultra-hominization."[36] This might be taken to suggest a narrative of transformation similar to that presented by many transhumanists: the passage into a higher state of spiritual existence by means of enhanced capacities for mental operations. Many of his fellow Christian theologians would find this notion hubristic, and rightly so. Such criticisms point to a major problem with the transhumanist worldview: the notion that death may be conquered and immortality gained by human effort alone.

In the Christian tradition, death is the final end of earthly life and the principal means by which God acts on the human person.[37] Teilhard accepts this fundamental truth of Christian existence in ways that his critics have typically failed to recognize. In an essay titled "The Death-Barrier and Co-Reflection," he considers the idea that humans will gain immortality by becoming incorporated into a reflective reality that will endure beyond the life span of their material body. It is true, he admits, that present-day humanity is the first generation to have enjoyed, in earthly life, this vision of what he calls ultrahumanity—"not only the promise of some millions of years of existence but a permanent immortality."[38] He nevertheless sees this possible earthly immortality as countered, on a phenomenological plane, by opposing forces of material decomposition. Indeed, in the ultrahuman context these forces are "vastly aggravated and amplified" by material decomposition, the powerful global vested interests that drive technological development, and the self-abnegation expected of the ordinary human workers on whose exertion progress depends.[39] Today, we might add that global warming is another major material factor limiting humankind's ability to gain immortality by technological effort.

Teilhard argues that belief in some kind of immortality is necessary to animate human action. The values and products of action must be believed to possess worth that endures beyond individual human lives.[40] Moreover, Teilhard reaffirms the classic Christian expectation of the future as being not senescence but immortality.[41] But he also makes clear in most of his writings that neither individual humans nor the human race collectively can circumvent death, even if spiritually transformed. It is precisely as a result of individual and collective death, he contends, that the "hominized essence of man may be released from, and continue to subsist outside of, the machinery of physical energies within which it developed."[42] Death, understood as the termination of physically embodied earthly life, is therefore unconquered by brands of transhumanism that posit the spiritual translation of humanity into a new sphere of existence.

What then of the transhumanist attempt to vanquish death not by spiritualization but by interventions to improve human bodies and cognitive capacities? These might be extremely high-technology interventions, or mundane but nevertheless revolutionary life choices in a matter such as diet, which is a key strand in Kurzweil's transhumanism. But Teilhard regards matter as intrinsically perishable and as dependent for its organization on spiritual principles. For this reason he would regard positively the shift in transhumanist interest from the enhancement of material life to the spiritualization of that life, although, as has been seen, would question the terms in which transhumanists usually understand this spiritualization.

Teilhard contemplated death close-up, as has Kurzweil. By the time he had reached the age of forty-five years, Teilhard had witnessed the deaths of six of his ten brothers and sisters, one of whom had been paralyzed by tuberculosis throughout most of her adult life.[43] Likewise, Kurzweil vividly describes the impact made on his life by the deaths of both his father and paternal grandfather from heart disease, and his subsequent successful efforts to improve his own physical health through diet and other measures after being diagnosed with diabetes.[44] Yet despite similar kinds of experience, these two thinkers perceive death in fundamentally different terms. Kurzweil presents death primarily as an obstacle to be overcome by ever-advancing ingenuity. Teilhard, in contrast, sees death as bearing transformative value, and even as giving human life its ultimate meaning. Indeed, death *is* spiritualization. Only by dying may humans escape universal entropy and enter a realm of assured convergence, synthesis, and unification.[45] Humans are transformed not in isolation, because essential to this transformation is union both with God and with other souls. Yet transformation is nevertheless fully individualized in the endings of specific personal human lives, as well as being part of a larger collective movement.

Transformation is ultimately due, therefore, to a cause subsisting beyond immanent earthly reality, but which nevertheless informs and transforms this reality. Evoking biblical descriptions of Jesus Christ appearing at the end of the world, Teilhard names this Omega: a point of attraction and transformation that is in essence individual, actual, and transcendent. It is individual insofar as it is identifiably part of earthly reality, in which the multiple complex centers and persons composing this reality participate. It is actual because it is a source of attraction, and thus acts upon these centers. Finally, it is transcendent, because it is "partly independent of the evolution that culminates in it."[46] Understanding development as a movement toward an active end point suggests that it should be seen as progression from a lack of being toward completion, not, as the transhumanists tend to picture it, as advancement from one point of self-sufficient plenitude to another.

This indicates that, for Teilhard, the Singularity is not finality. However unimaginably spectacular or rapid the world's reflective transformation might be, there remains a point of transformation at which humans cease to transform the world by acting on it and begin to be transformed by the action on them of a superior agent. For Kurzweil and the other transhumanists, in contrast, the Singularity does not have a superior origin and is therefore not strictly transcendent. By denying the possibility of any real transcendence, they offer an image of humanity imprisoned within a time-bound universe. Their dematerialized spiritualism is, as discussed above, the product of a strange confluence of a type of Christian theology that undervalued the material, embodied dimension of human life with a secular ideology of progress achieved as a result of human effort alone.

Teilhard shares the concern expressed by many of the transhumanists about concepts of God that seem to have been developed either to curtail human development or to resolve difficult questions surrounding the nature of human existence such as what happens after death. Yet by denying the possibility of a transcendent infinite acting on humans, the transhumanists deny to finite humanity the very infinite end they seek to attain for them. To see human creativity, as do the transhumanists, as intimating infinity, it is unnecessary to regard such ingenuity as eliminating or replacing this infinity. On the contrary, as Austin Farrer argues, humans grasp the notion of infinity through, in, and as creative activity—and indeed are able to grasp it in no other way.[47] Furthermore, from a theological perspective, this vision of the absolute manifesting itself in and through transformative but ultimately finite activity is vastly preferable to attempts to understand God directly, which inevitably objectivize and relativize an ultimately unknowable cause.[48] So by being receptive to some transhumanist ideas, theologians might even find ways of addressing some of their own problems.

This analogical understanding of the finity–infinity relation is entirely compatible with the promotion of human creativity and industry. Indeed, such an understanding is essential in order to conceive humankind's truly infinite dimension, rather than consigning it to a bleak everlasting finitude that is merely proportionate with its current mode of existence. If human life is to be meaningful, it ultimately needs contingency, change, and decay to be made ready for real transformation. The transhumanist vision of everlasting earthly life, which is symptomatic of a failure of the Christian analogical imagination, seeks to replace these capacities for radical openness to divine action with a bland uniformity that would make life meaningless. But as the Gospels show us, it is in a life lived in the face of finitude, suffering, and finally death—however painful or undeserved these might be—where true transformation and transcendence are to be found.

Notes

1. Bostrom, "History of Transhumanist Thought," 10.
2. Steinhart, "Teilhard de Chardin."
3. Teilhard de Chardin, *Future of Man*, 297.
4. Huxley, "Transhumanism."
5. Cuénot, *Teilhard de Chardin*, 302–6.
6. Teilhard de Chardin, *Man's Place in Nature*, 32–36.
7. Kurzweil, *Singularity*, 40–50; Kurzweil, *Age of Spiritual Machines*, 14.
8. Teilhard de Chardin, *Man's Place in Nature*, 72–78.
9. Kurzweil, *Singularity*, 487.
10. Teilhard de Chardin, *Future of Man*, 228–31; Bostrom, "Future of Humanity," 191.
11. Teilhard de Chardin, *Future of Man*, 276–77.
12. Kurzweil, *Singularity*, 20–21.
13. Teilhard de Chardin, *Man's Place*, 110.

14. Teilhard de Chardin, *Future of Man*, 155–84; Kurzweil, *Age of Spiritual Machines*, 171.

15. Teilhard de Chardin, *Toward the Future*, 183–84; Teilhard de Chardin, *Human Phenomenon*, 122–23; Teilhard de Chardin, *Future of Man*, 166.

16. Kurzweil, *Singularity*, 7, 14–21.

17. Teilhard de Chardin, *Toward the Future*, 181.

18. Bostrom, "Human Genetic Enhancements," 493.

19. Teilhard de Chardin, *Future of Man*, 182–84.

20. Grumett, "Teilhard de Chardin's Evolutionary Natural Theology," 530.

21. Teilhard de Chardin, *Activation of Energy*, 237.

22. Ibid., 306.

23. Teilhard de Chardin, *Future of Man*, 170–71.

24. Teilhard de Chardin, *Divine Milieu*.

25. Teilhard de Chardin, *Toward the Future*, 102–6.

26. Grumett, *Teilhard de Chardin*, 238.

27. Murdoch, *Metaphysics as a Guide to Morals*, 511.

28. Bostrom and Ćirković, "Introduction," 27.

29. Teilhard de Chardin, *Christianity and Evolution*, 23.

30. Teilhard de Chardin, *Future of Man*, 202.

31. Ibid., *Man*, 204.

32. Bostrom and Sandberg, "Wisdom of Nature," at 396–97.

33. Ibid., 398–405.

34. Teilhard de Chardin, *Future of Man*, 234.

35. Teilhard de Chardin, *Activation*, 307.

36. Ibid., 380.

37. Nichols, "Radical Life Extension."

38. Teilhard de Chardin, *Activation*, 399.

39. Ibid., 400.

40. Ibid., 41, 334.

41. Teilhard de Chardin, *Future of Man*, 295.

42. Teilhard de Chardin, *Activation*, 138.

43. Grumett, *Teilhard de Chardin*, 77–78.

44. Kurzweil and Grossman, *Fantastic Voyage*, 33–34, 139.

45. Teilhard de Chardin, *Human Phenomenon*, 194.

46. Teilhard de Chardin, *Activation*, 112–13.

47. Farrer, *Finite and Infinite*, 26.

48. Ibid., 37.

References

Bostrom, Nick. "The Future of Humanity." In *New Waves in Philosophy of Technology*, edited by Jan Kyrre Berg Olsen, Evan Selinger, and Søren Riis. New York: Palgrave Macmillan, 2009.

———. "A History of Transhumanist Thought." *Journal of Evolution and Technology* 14 (2005): 1–25.

———. "Human Genetic Enhancements: A Transhumanist Perspective." *Journal of Value Enquiry* 37 (2003): 493–506.

Bostrom, Nick, and Milan M. Ćirković. "Introduction." In *Global Catastrophic Risks*, edited by Nick Bostrom and Milan M. Ćirković. New York: Oxford University Press, 2008.

Bostrom, Nick, and Anders Sandberg. "The Wisdom of Nature: An Evolutionary Heuristic for Human Enhancement." In *Human Enhancement*, edited by Julian Savulescu and Nick Bostrom. New York: Oxford University Press, 2009.

Cuénot, Claude. *Teilhard de Chardin: A Biographical Study.* London: Burns & Oates, 1965.

Farrer, Austin. *Finite and Infinite: A Philosophical Essay.* London: Dacre, 1943.

Grumett, David. "Teilhard de Chardin's Evolutionary Natural Theology." *Zygon* 42 (2007): 519–34.

———. *Teilhard de Chardin: Theology, Humanity and Cosmos.* Leuven: Peeters, 2005.

Huxley, Julian. "Transhumanism." In *New Bottles for New Wine: Essays.* London: Chatto & Windus, 1957.

Kurzweil, Ray. *The Age of Spiritual Machines: How We Will Live, Work and Think in the New Age of Intelligent Machines.* New York: Viking Press, 1999.

———. *The Singularity Is Near: When Humans Transcend Biology.* New York: Viking Press, 2005.

Kurzweil, Raymond, and Terry Grossman. *Fantastic Voyage: Live Long Enough to Live Forever.* Emmaus, PA: Rodale Press, 2004.

Murdoch, Iris. *Metaphysics as a Guide to Morals.* New York: Penguin, 1993.

Nichols, Terence L. "Radical Life Extension: Implications for Roman Catholicism." In *Religion and the Implications of Radical Life Extension*, edited by Derek F. Maher, Calvin Mercer, and Ted Peters. New York: Palgrave Macmillan, 2009.

Steinhart, Eric. "Teilhard de Chardin and Transhumanism." *Journal of Evolution and Technology* 20 (2008): 1–22.

Teilhard de Chardin, Pierre. *Activation of Energy*, translated by Reneì Hague. San Diego: Harvest, 1978.

———. *Christianity and Evolution*, translated by René Hague. New York : Harcourt Brace Jovanovich,1971.

———. *The Divine Milieu*, translated by Siôn Cowell. Portland: Sussex Academic Press, 2003.

———. *The Future of Man*, translated by Norman Denny. New York: Harper & Row, 1964.

———. *The Human Phenomenon*, translated by Sarah Appleton-Weber. Portland: Sussex Academic Press, 2003.

———. *Man's Place in Nature: The Human Zoological Group*, translated by René Hague. New York: Harper & Row, 1966.

———. *Toward the Future*, translated by René Hague. San Diego: Harvest, 1975.

Chapter Four

Dignity and Enhancement in the Holy City

KAREN LEBACQZ

The enhancement debate appears as an "either/or"—*either* enhancement threatens something about our human dignity because it defies limits intrinsic to human beings and hence to human dignity, *or* enhancement may contribute to human dignity. The first is roughly the view of the President's Council on Bioethics in *Beyond Therapy*; the second is a position expressed by Nick Bostrom in his critique of that volume.[1] I propose that, from a Christian perspective, the impact of enhancement on human dignity need not be an "either/or." Rather, there are reasons both to offer some cautions and also to affirm many if not most enhancements to human life.

The more interesting question may be: What constitutes a genuine "enhancement," and of what does "dignity" consist? For purposes of this chapter I accept Bostrom's definition of an enhancement as an intervention that "improves the functioning of some subsystem of an organism beyond its reference state" or "creates an entirely new functioning or subsystem that the organism previously lacked."[2] By "reference state," Bostrom intends the "normal, healthy" state of a subsystem. The meaning of dignity is itself a controversial topic, and some hints toward an understanding will emerge as we proceed.

The Debate

The President's Council on Bioethics, in *Beyond Therapy*, offers the view that, as tempting as some "enhancements" may be, they are dangerous and should be avoided because they threaten something important about human dignity. For example, with regard to the question of using enhancements in sports, the council asserts that "understanding the true dignity of excellent human activity" will show us that "new ways of improving performance may distort or undermine it."[3] To support this position the council points out that the dignity of a sport is determined not by the *result* but by the *way* it is done and by the identity of the doer. A runner on steroids, they suggest, is less obviously "himself" and less obviously "human" than is his opponent who has not taken steroids. In short the act done must be a "human" act—it must be truly "one's own." Only then, the council implies, does it exhibit human dignity.

But what about the fact that we are *choosing* animals? If choosing makes us distinctively human, then why is the choice of using steroids not precisely a manifestation of human dignity? The answer to this question given by the President's Council on Bioethics is carefully nuanced: The problem lies not in the choosing per se, but in the fact that we have chosen to bypass our bodily integrity.[4] In so doing, we have "divided" ourselves and have ceased to be an embodied unity. Hence, our dignity must reside to some degree in accepting our embodiment and honoring the limits that it places on us. Our excellence must be our own embodied excellence; only then can it be considered dignified. "What matters is that we produce the given result . . . in a human way as human beings, not simply as inputs who produce out-puts."[5] In short the council asserts that there is a difference between "real" and "false" excellence. It is *human agency* that gives superior performance its dignity.[6]

These reflections on human agency and its role in human dignity are given an even stronger emphasis in the summary to *Beyond Therapy*. Here, the President's Council on Bioethics asserts that the Promethean tempta-tion to remake nature is to be faulted not simply because it may lead to bad consequences but also because it is a wrong attitude: It is a failure to appreciate and respect the "given-ness" or "giftedness" of the world.[7] What is disquieting about the use of drugs to improve memory or alertness is not that such drugs are artificial; after all, medicine itself is artificial in that sense. The real issue is the problem of self-alienation.[8] There may be human goods that are inseparable from our aging bodies, for example.[9] Living with full awareness of our finitude may be the condition of the best things in human life—engagement, seriousness, a taste for beauty, the quest for meaning, and so on. The council asserts: "A flourishing human life is not a life lived with an ageless body or an untroubled soul, but rather a life lived in rhythmed time, mindful of time's limits."[10] In our enhancement efforts, we risk making our bodies and minds little more than tools, turning into "someone else," flat-tening our souls, and ignoring the pursuit of true happiness. In short, to bor-row a phrase from Bostrom, the council believes that enhancement efforts will threaten our human dignity by "clipping the wings of our souls."[11]

It is ironic that this phrase comes from Bostrom, given that he takes issue with the President's Council on Bioethics and its resistant stance toward enhancement. He argues that "enhancement" might indeed *increase* a cer-tain *kind* of dignity—namely, "dignity as a quality." He first proposes a "tax-onomy" of dignity: dignity as a quality or kind of excellence; simple human dignity (*Menshenwurde*), which relates to the full moral status of humans; and dignity as social status, which is a relational property admitting of gradations.[12] Then, drawing on Aurel Kolnai, Bostrom defines dignity as a quality as a kind of "worthiness" on a par with basic moral virtues. In this sense, dignity is a "thick" moral concept—both descriptive and evaluative. It calls for a response of respect.

What are the qualities that lead to such a response? Using Kolnai again, Bostrom proposes: composure, calm, restraint, reserve, and distinctness, a sense of being invulnerable, inaccessible to destructive or corruptive influence.[13] As Kolnai says, "the dignified quietly defies the world."[14] Bostrom summarizes dignity as a quality with the phrase "dignified inner equilibrium."[15]

Dignified inner equilibrium implies maintaining composure under stress. What if that composure is maintained because we took a pill such as Paxil? Does the *method* used to attain composure matter to our dignity? Surely we want composure to be part of an *authentic* response. Does taking an "enhancement" pill make it less authentic? The President's Council on Bioethics would probably say yes. Bostrom says no; a capacity that is or becomes ours because we *chose* it is at least as authentically ours as a capacity that we are simply "born with."[16] In 1486, Pico della Mirandola, in *Oration on the Dignity of Man*, noted that humans are not determined by laws of nature. He therefore proffered the view that our dignity consists in our capacity for self-shaping. "It is thus possible to argue that the act of voluntary, deliberate enhancement *adds* to the dignity of the resulting trait, compared to possessing the same trait by mere default," declares Bostrom.[17] In other words, his point is that the deliberate use of "enhancements" such as drugs *might* improve the functioning that allows qualities of dignity such as composure and distinctness to be exhibited. Of course, some enhancements might not do so; but if any *can* do so, then we cannot say that enhancement per se threatens human dignity. Rather, we must allow the possibility that the deliberate use of enhancement techniques such as drugs can contribute to human dignity.

However, another challenge remains. For Leon Kass, who chaired the President's Council on Bioethics during the time when *Beyond Therapy* was prepared, it is not simply a question of whether certain traits associated with dignity can be maintained or improved by "enhancement." Kass suggests that there are *two* paths to undignity: (1) We might choose the *wrong traits* to enhance; or (2) the very *process* of refashioning ourselves may reduce our dignity.[18] It is the second path that is of particular concern to Kass and to the council: Does the very process of self-transformation yield a less dignified human being?

Bostrom tackles this question as well. Deliberate self-transformation might be dignity-enhancing or dignity-reducing, he asserts.[19] Drawing again on Kolnai, he argues that the *motivation* for enhancement may matter. Enhancements that are driven by "alien" wants or that represent surrender to mere convenience are not dignified—for example, enhancing our cognition because we are taken in by slick advertising. The enhanced cognition may appear to be a gain in dignity, but something has nonetheless been lost by how we achieved it, because it was not an authentic choice. (Thus, choice can be deliberate without being authentic.) By implication, Bostrom here appears to agree with the council that if we are simply taking the "easy way out," we are reducing our dignity. There is, then, some common ground between them. Where they differ may be at the point where Bostrom notes that choosing *not* to "enhance" ourselves may be undignified, whereas for the council remaining within our given limits lends us dignity.[20]

What about modifications of our affective responses? In *Brave New World*, which figures rather prominently in Kass's work, Aldous Huxley has given us a prototypical image of undignity: The drug "soma" reduces people to contented but unimaginative citizen-blobs instead of individuals. Another prototypical image is the rat wired to press a lever that simply induces a state of pleasure; surrendering to the induced pleasure state, the rat stops eating, striving, and so on. Such images of undignity suggest that dignity as a quality must include "a controlled passion for life and what it has to offer," says Bostrom.[21] To be rendered devoid of emotion would be to lose dignity. If being "well-adjusted" means losing our ideals and our capacity to respond with the full register of human emotion, then we have lost dignity, in Bostrom's view. Indeed, he suggests in subsequent sections that Western culture has already lost a great deal of "dignity as a quality."[22] Loss of passion or emotion or striving would constitute a loss of human dignity. People could use emotional enhancements to "clip the wings of their own souls."

Hence dignity seems to require a certain level of passion for life. Emotions matter. At the same time, to be dignified, our emotions also need to be "appropriate responses to aspects of the world."[23] Bostrom does not make reference here to the classic virtue of prudence, but one might easily extend his argument in this direction; prudence is the virtue of acting in accord with the real.[24] Human dignity, then, is indeed related to classic virtues—it requires passion and energy appropriately tailored to the demands of the situation.

Bostrom also considers whether creatures or things besides humans might have "dignity as a quality"—for example, elephants or redwood trees. He uses Stephen Darwall's distinction between "recognition respect," giving appropriate consideration, and "appraisal respect," an attitude of positive appraisal.[25] When we say that human dignity must be respected, we are talking about recognition respect. Dignity as a quality, however, seems to be about appraisal respect—it is something possessed by only some agents. Redwood trees or elephants must be given recognition respect, but not appraisal respect—that is, we do not have to give credit to them for having grown so tall or being so strong.

Finally, Bostrom calls dignity as a quality one of the "quiet values," as compared with the "loud values" of suffering, justice, or freedom.[26] The loud values will almost always trump the quiet values, but over time the quiet values are terribly important, he argues; they "add the luminescence, the rich texture of meaning, the wonder and awe, and much of the beauty and nobility of human action."[27] Hence, in a futuristic "Plastic World" (posthuman) of superintelligent inhabitants who have complete power over and understanding of themselves and control of their environment, and where the loud values have been resolved, the quiet values will become more important, and it is by accepting some constraints on their actions that these future inhabitants will preserve their dignity as a quality.[28]

In spite of their seeming differences, then, both sides of this debate appear to concur on several matters. Specifically, they concur that enhancement *can* threaten dignity, and that the preservation of dignity has something to do with the *way* in which things are done and with keeping them preeminently human. Where they differ is with regard to bodily limits. For Kass and the President's Council on Bioethics, bodily limits must be honored for humans to have dignity. For Bostrom, bodily limits themselves do not determine human dignity and need not be honored; rather, dignity resides in the choosing capacities of humans and how those capacities are exercised.

A Christian Response

What might be a Christian response to this disagreement? In its many permutations, Christian theology is at root a "Creation–Fall–Redemption" theology. Although Christian denominations differ in their emphases, all work from a basic story of God's good creation that has been distorted but is then "redeemed" by God. Within this story, many themes related to the Creation and Fall evoke the notion that limits should be set on human striving and hence, possibly, on enhancement efforts. The question, then, is what it means for the fallen world to be "redeemed" and whether such redemption might surpass the cautions present in the Creation and Fall scenarios; what would an emphasis on Redemption bring to the question of encompassing enhancements? Here I argue that Redemption trumps Creation and Fall and therefore permits some latitude for enhancement.

Cautions

At the outset, however, it must be acknowledged that the Bible is full of cautionary tales encouraging us to know and accept limits to human striving. First among these are the two creation stories. Both Genesis 1 and Genesis 2:5–9 emphasize that humans are not God; we are *creature* rather than *Creator*. God created humans and breathed life into them and placed them in the Garden of Eden. We may be made in the "image" of God (Gen 1:26–27), but this does not mean that we *are* God. Indeed, some theologians interpret the "image of God" to mean that we are a mere "reflection" of God's glory.[29] Image and original are not the same; to "reflect" God's light or creativity is not the same as being the source of light or creativity. Our role is to be stewards of God's good creation. Power and control remain with God, and any effort to claim the power of creation over ourselves is seen as "playing God" and brings with it condemnation. These concerns are common in Christian theology. Creation alone seems to set some limits on what we may do.

Added to those limits are cautions deriving from the Christian affirmation that we live in a "fallen" world—a world distorted from God's original intentions. God's original creation was "very good" (Gen 1:30), and the Garden of Eden was intended to give humans everything needed for a good life. But humans disobeyed God's commandments, and as a result were evicted from the Garden of Eden and condemned to live with strife, hard work, and death (Gen 3:14–19).[30] Having been evicted from the Garden of Eden, humans no longer even know clearly what God's intentions are; thus, we are always in danger of substituting our own judgment for that of God. This danger should give us pause before we attempt to "re-create" ourselves.

The story of Noah and the Great Flood is another cautionary tale. Seeing how much evil humans had done, God regretted creating them and determined to wipe them off the face of the Earth (Gen 6:5–7). But Noah was a righteous man, so God permitted Noah to build an ark in order to escape the coming flood. Noah and his family survived, and after the flood God made a new covenant with Noah. In this covenant, God promised never again to curse the very ground because of the sins of humankind (Gen 8:21), but God also stipulated that humans must henceforth be accountable for the "life blood" of other humans and other creatures. It is this precise passage that Leon Kass interprets to provide some grounding for asserting that our very "blood" and hence, our embodiment, must be taken to set some limits on human aspirations.[31]

Finally, there is the story of the Tower of Babel (Gen 11:1–9). Using bricks and mortar, the people of the earth decided to build a city with a tower that reached into the heavens. God was not pleased with the idea that "henceforward, nothing they have a mind to do will be beyond their reach" (Gen 11:6). The "confusion" of languages that God imposed at Babel is precisely intended to keep the people from reaching too far into the heavens. In other words, we are to stay "on the ground" and not try to reach "Heaven," the domain of God. We must live within our limits.

These are not the only biblical tales that might be seen as cautionary, but they provide a sufficient framework for explaining why many who are informed by biblical stories and themes hesitate to embrace any human act that appears to defy natural limits. All these stories suggest that we must be ever mindful of hubris, of overreaching and trying to go "beyond" our humanness. Thus there are reasons to offer cautions about "enhancements," as do Kass and the President's Council on Bioethics. In a Christian vision, it is not our place to "play God" or to replace God's plan for us; rather, as stewards of the life we have been given by God, it is our task to preserve God's values and intentions to the best of our ability.

Affirmations

What are the values and intentions that are entrusted to our stewardship? Must stewardship be limited to preserving what *is*? Many theologians think not. If God is the Creator, and we are created in God's image, then are we not also meant to create? The Lutheran Philip Hefner and the Methodist Lynn Rhodes have both used the image of "cocreators" to express the sense that being made in the image of God *includes* the idea that we are not simply "creatures" but also creators.[32]

The stories of Jesus's actions on Earth may be taken to suggest the overcoming of limits. Healing stories certainly play a central role in depictions of Jesus's life and ministry. But some would say these show only that we are meant to attain the "normal, healthy" functioning of human life and not to go beyond it. If such stories never go beyond our natural limits, then they hardly suggest support for enhancement efforts. Is there any evidence in these stories of genuine *transcendence* of human life and limits or enhancement beyond the simple restoration of health?

I believe so. Setting aside ultimate resurrection,[33] we might look at the story of Jesus raising Lazarus from the dead (Jn 11:1–44).[34] This story at a minimum suggests transcendence of the most crucial limit on human life, which is death. Further, the Gospels are full of stories where water is turned to wine or a few loaves and fishes feed thousands. Can there be any doubt that, in these stories, normal limits have been set aside? Nor are these acts limited to Jesus's behavior; the disciples are also meant to do such "miracles" (Rom 8:14). These stories suggest at a minimum that ordinary human limits can be overcome. Indeed, one might say that it is in the overcoming of such ordinary limits that we see, preeminently, God's intentions manifest among us.

"I have come that [people] may have life and may have it in all its fullness," says Jesus in the Gospel of John (Jn 10:10). The intention of abundant life or *fullness of life* is central to God's promises to us.[35] The image of abundant life has become a powerful vehicle for Christian theology.[36] If God's desire for our fullness of life and God's promise of this fullness constitute the *telos* toward which we are moving, then it is not clear that enhancements should be resisted. Anything that "improves" our life and makes it "fuller" may be countenanced.

Indeed, in *God: The World's Future—Systematic Theology for a New Era*, Ted Peters argues precisely that creation stories must be read in the light of God's intentions for fullness of life.[37] The God of our future salvation, suggests Peters, is not limited by what already exists. God creates "from the future." God's constant work is future giving. When we look at the stories of creation, therefore, we must read them in the light of God's ultimate purposes, revealed in God's redemptive work. The image of God, then, is a constant call *forward*. Peters calls it "the divine draw toward future reality."[38] Becoming fully human, then, is a not a return to some state of origin or to the old creation; it is a "future arrival for the first time."[39] Our true humanity is *eschatological*.

The future toward which God draws us is imaged in the final book of the Bible, the Book of Revelation. Revelation attests to our transcendence of any limits set in the Garden of Eden and the "Fall." In the last chapters of Revelation (21–22), a "new Heaven and Earth" are described. In this new Heaven and Earth there is a "Holy City," in which "there shall be no more death. . . . . Neither shall there be any more pain: For the former things are passed away" (21:4b). "All things" are made new (21:5).[40] If "all things" are made new, this must include human beings ourselves, and thus there is reason to embrace enhancement that takes away pain, death, and limits on human life. We are *meant* to transcend our limits, to draw close to God, to live in the "Holy City" described in the Book of Revelation.[41] Doing so does not threaten our dignity but rather expresses precisely what our human destiny and dignity are intended to be—a life of abundance (the streets are of gold, the walls of jasper, and the foundation stones of emeralds and other precious jewels), in which all are included (the gates of the city are never shut), all are fed (the river of the water of life flows down the middle, with trees that yield fruit every month of the year and whose leaves heal the nations), God dwells at ease among the people (there is no more temple, one can finally "see the face of God and live"), and all "accursed things" disappear.

Concluding Unscientific Postscript

The image of transcendence presented in the Book of Revelation also raises interesting questions as to the *content* of enhancement and of dignity. Both the President's Council on Bioethics and Nick Bostrom, in his reflections on quiet values, appear to assume that accepting some limits will be a necessary part of *true* human dignity. The council would have us accept these limits now, before we begin any serious program of enhancement. Bostrom would allow us to get to a "Plastic World" but then believes that with all the loud values under control, the quiet values would begin to emerge as central to human dignity. Both seem to believe that at some point, the true essence of human dignity lies in accepting some limits and not working toward every enhancement. Does the image of the Holy City in the book of Revelation support such a view?

This is a difficult question to answer, especially for one who is not a biblical scholar. Certainly, on the sheer face of the text, it would appear that loud values such as justice are completely "in hand" in the Holy City—a river of life feeds all the people, none are outside the gate, and so on. Justice seems to reign. Further, ease of life seems to be the norm; as precious gems abound, the text carries the connotation that all are not simply fed but are indeed rich. What, then, of those quiet values of restraint, modesty, and such that are often associated with "dignity as a quality"? Is it in these that true dignity lies? Boldly, I want to suggest that it is not. Rather, the text implies that humans may finally stand "face to face" with God. We do, indeed, become more than human, other than human, or humans as we are ultimately meant to be—creatures, yes, but creatures who can "see the face of God and live." We have transcended the limits set in the Garden of Eden. This vision of the destiny of humans suggests that, although we should always remember our current fallen state and tendency toward hubris, we need not at root fear enhancements—it is our destiny to be more than we were at creation, to become friends with God and partners in the Holy City. Our very dignity may lie in our transcendence of limits and in our orientation toward that eschatological call from God. We have reason to proceed with some cautions, given our current fallen state, but we also have reason to proceed with trust and hope, given our future vocation.

Notes

1. President's Council on Bioethics, *Beyond Therapy*; Bostrom, "Dignity and Enhancement."
2. Ibid., 179.
3. President's Council on Bioethics, *Beyond Therapy*, 140–45.

4. Ibid.,147ff.

5. Ibid., 153.

6. Ibid., 155.

7. Ibid., 288.

8. Ibid., 294.

9. Ibid., 296. The council notes that this insight is "counterintuitive." The passage is therefore crucial, for it suggests that what the council takes to be "dignity" will not always accord with what appears most obviously to be the value or "worth" of human life.

10. President's Council on Bioethics, *Beyond Therapy*, 299.

11. Bostrom, "Dignity," 191.

12. Ibid., 175–78.

13. Two good examples of such "dignity as a quality" might be Nelson Mandela during his years in prison and the character played by Morgan Freeman in the film *Driving Miss Daisy*. Both maintained composure and a sense of being incorruptible in spite of oppression and treatment that was both unjust and demeaning. Womanist theologian Katie Canon speaks of the "invisible dignity" of the oppressed.

14. Quoted by Bostrom, "Dignity," 179. Kolnai apparently also considered cats to be dignified!

15. Ibid., 180.

16. Ibid., 182.

17. Ibid., 184.

18. Ibid., 185.

19. Ibid., 186.

20. Ibid., 187.

21. Ibid., 189.

22. However, he notes that attributing dignity as a quality to cultures or civilizations relies more heavily on value judgments than attributing it to individuals. Ibid., 193.

23. Ibid., 190.

24. Pieper, *Four Cardinal Virtues*, 10.

25. Bostrom, "Dignity," 199.

26. Ibid., 200.

27. Ibid., 201.

28. Ibid., 203. In his critique of Bostrom, Charles Rubin argues that Bostrom misuses Kolnai; see Rubin, "Commentary on Bostrom," 207–11. "According to Kolnai, true dignity (and its opposite) arises only in how we come to terms with things not of our own choice or making." Thus, genuine human dignity requires accepting "certain natural necessities," Rubin argues. Though Bostrom suggests that the "quiet values" would become more important in "plastic world," Rubin argues that there is nothing in Bostrom's plastic world that would induce its inhabitants to show self-restraint. I concur; Bostrom seems, ironically, to want to agree with Kass that self-restraint is a necessary part of "dignity" for humans, yet there is nothing in his argument to demonstrate why this should be so.

29. R. Kendall Soulen and Linda Woodhead write: "Glory is not a natural human endowment; it is the reflection of the light of God." Soulen and Woodhead, "Introduction," 24.

30. It is particularly interesting that the commandment disobeyed here is that commandment not to eat of the tree of the "knowledge of good and evil." In other words, it is precisely our ethical efforts that occasion the "fall." Note that Holmes Rolston takes as one of the defining characteristics of human dignity our capacity to be ethical beings. Rolston, "Human Uniqueness," 148ff.

31. Kass, "Defending Human Dignity," 323.

32. Hefner, "Evolution of the Created Co-Creator"; Rhodes, Co-Creating.

33. Christian belief in the resurrection is a preeminent place of transcendence of the primary limit of human life, which is death. But is resurrection only for Jesus; does it apply to those of us who are not "fully god?" Is it only for the "end times" with no relevance for the here and now? Theological interpretations of the resurrection are legion and problematic, and I cannot resolve such questions fully here. Some, for example, would say that resurrection comes only at the very "end" of time and cannot apply to life on earth here and now. Therefore, I ignore ultimate resurrection here.

34. "Raising from the dead" may not be the equivalent of resurrection, since those "raised from the dead" will die again. This claim is argued by Rick Reinckens at www.godonthe.net/evidence/Lazarus.htm. James Merrill Hamilton notes that this story is missing from the Synoptic Gospels and this has raised questions as to the authenticity of the recorded event; see www.bible.org/page.php?page_id=2049. But also see the parallel stories in Mt 9:18–26, Mk 5:41–42, and Lk 8:52–56 and 7:11–15. For my purposes, however, it is not crucial whether such stores are historically true but only that they illustrate a particular mindset of overcoming normal human limits.

35. See Peters, Lebacqz, and Bennett, Sacred Cells?

36. E.g., see McFague, Life Abundant; and Day and Dykstra, For Life Abundant. There are also churches that operate under the rubric of "Abundant Life" congregations.

37. Peters, God.

38. Ibid., 147.

39. Ibid., 156.

40. Interestingly, in the Holy City, there is no temple, as the presence of God simply permeates everything; also, people will finally be able to see the face of God and live.

41. Of course, the Book of Revelation belongs to the biblical literature called "apocalyptic," and proper interpretation of that literature has been controversial. Here, I assume that we are given not a literal reading of the future but an image to organize our lives. Perhaps most controversial is the question of whether humans can bring about this "new Heaven and Earth" or whether we must wait for God to do so. In the tradition that stresses our cocreation with God, I assume it is a "both-and" endeavor.

References

Bostrom, Nick. "Dignity and Enhancement." In *Human Dignity and Bioethics: Essays Commissioned by the President's Council*, edited by President's Council on Bioethics. Washington, DC: US Government Printing Office, 2008. http://bioethics.georgetown.edu/pcbe/reports/human_dignity/human_dignity_and _bioethics.pdf.

Day, Dorothy C., and Craig Dykstra, eds. *For Life Abundant: Practical Theology, Theological Education, and Christian Ministry*. Grand Rapids: William B. Eerdmans, 2008.

Hefner, Philip. "The Evolution of the Created Co-Creator." In *Cosmos as Creation: Science and Theology in Consonance*, edited by Ted Peters. Nashville: Abingdon Press, 1989.

Kass, Leon. "Defending Human Dignity." In *Human Dignity and Bioethics: Essays Commissioned by the President's Council*, edited by President's Council on Bioethics. Washington, DC: US Government Printing Office, 2008. http://bioethics.georgetown.edu/pcbe/reports/human_dignity/human_dignity_and _bioethics.pdf.

McFague, Sallie. *Life Abundant: Rethinking Theology and Economy for a Planet in Peril*. Minneapolis: Fortress Press, 2000.

Peters, Ted. *God: The World's Future—Systematic Theology for a New Era*, 2nd ed. Minneapolis: Fortress Press, 2000.

Peters, Ted, Karen Lebacqz, and Gaymon Bennett. *Sacred Cells? Why Christians Should Support Stem Cell Research*. Lanham, MD: Rowman & Littlefield, 2008.

Pieper, Josef. *The Four Cardinal Virtues: Prudence, Justice, Fortitude, Temperance*, translated by Richard Winston. Notre Dame: University of Notre Dame, 1966.

President's Council on Bioethics. *Beyond Therapy: Biotechnology and the Pursuit of Happiness*. New York: HarperCollins, 2003. http://bioethics.georgetown.edu/ pcbe/reports/beyondtherapy/beyond_therapy_final_webcorrected.pdf.

Rhodes, Lynn N. *Co-Creating: A Feminist Vision of Ministry*. Philadelphia: Westminster Press, 1987.

Rolston, Holmes, III. "Human Uniqueness and Human Dignity." In *Human Dignity and Bioethics: Essays Commissioned by the President's Council*, edited by President's Council on Bioethics. Washington, DC: US Government Printing Office, 2008. http://bioethics.georgetown.edu/pcbe/reports/human_dignity/human_ dignity_and_bioethics.pdf.

Rubin, Charles. "Commentary on Bostrom." In *Human Dignity and Bioethics: Essays Commissioned by the President's Council*, edited by President's Council on Bioethics. Washington, DC: US Government Printing Office, 2008. http://bioethics.georgetown.edu/pcbe/reports/human_dignity/human_dignity_and _bioethics.pdf.

Soulen, R. Kendall, and Linda Woodhead, eds. "Introduction." In *God and Human Dignity*. Grand Rapids: William B. Eerdmans, 2006.

Chapter Five

Progress and Provolution

Will Transhumanism Leave Sin Behind?

TED PETERS

"I like new things," my mother said one day during my youth. She was sitting on the sofa, running her hand over the upholstery and feeling the texture. The sofa was brand new. It had just been delivered by the department store. My mother did not experience such new things very frequently. This was a special day.

My father, in contrast, worked daily in the world of the new. He was an engineer for General Motors. Each day he awoke, dressed, and drove to work with the express intention of inventing something new—a gadget that hitherto had never existed in the history of the world. He finished his professional career with his name on twenty-two patents. Now my dad simply thought he was earning a living. He did not think often about the ontological implications of the new, the *novum*.

The theologian Jürgen Moltmann believes that the capacity of nature and history to experience the new and invent the new comes from God. God's creation is ever changing; and we as God's creatures have the capacity to accelerate and direct the course of this change. To attune ourselves to the God of the new, says Moltmann, we should open ourselves to the possibility of a transformative future, and we thus should adopt a "provolutionary" mindset: "In provolution, the human 'dream turned forward' is combined with the new possibility of the future and begins consciously to direct the course of human history as well as the evolution of nature."[1] Provolution is prompted by God's promise of eschatological transformation; and this promise inspires transformative human creativity. Evolution in nature can be extended and enhanced through distinctively human creativity.

The transhumanists and posthumanists among us exude the provolutionary spirit. Like runway lights guiding a pilot to the airport, the vision of the *novum* guides technoenthusiasts toward a future with a new kind of human being. Tomorrow's human being will be regeneticized, nanotechized, cyborgized, and perhaps even immortalized. Genetic science hybridized with nanotechnology and robotics will carry modern medicine well beyond our current occupation with healing the sick. In the next generation we will devise bodily systems that avoid disease, enhance our capacities, and qualitatively improve our physical and intellectual well-being.

The transhumanist vision includes immortality. Two roads might lead to overcoming death, one via the body and the other via the mind. First, perhaps with just the right genetic selection and genetic engineering, our enhanced physical health may make us immune to aging and ward off the diseases that might kill us prematurely. We will live forever (unless we get run over by a truck) in our bodies. But if this fails, second, technogeniuses might find a way to upload our brain capacity, including our self-consciousness, into a computer. Then, in our minds, we could live forever as software within computer hardware. We could sustain our immortality just as long as someone backs up our aging computer, of course.

What I like about the technoenthusiasts among us is the unapologetic extravagance of their vision. I like their zeal for transformation. I like their celebration of the new. Without knowing it, they are manifesting an important dimension of the image of God (*imago Dei*) within our civilization: the dimension of creativity and transformativity.

Yet a level of naïveté here risks a loss of realism. Good physical health, increased intelligence, and even the immortality of either the body or the mind would constitute a transformation, to be sure. It would mark a change. It would mark progress. It would lead to something new. And yet an item of looming significance is missing from this vision: a realistic appreciation for the depth and pervasiveness of what theologians call *sin*. As sinful creatures, we humans never lose our capacity to tarnish what is shiny, to undo what has been done, to corrupt what is pure.

As a theologian I ask: On the one hand, how can we appreciate and even encourage the inventiveness of our medical scientists and nanotechnologists while, on the other hand, we draw upon theological wisdom regarding human nature to tailor our expectations with human sinfulness in mind? How can we hope for change through human creativity while being realistic about what can and cannot be changed? How can we fuel technological and medical progress while recognizing that the ultimate human transformation—the ultimate provolution—will come as an act of divine grace?

As I begin to address these questions, I start where I find Ronald Cole-Turner and Celia Deane-Drummond. Cole-Turner alerts us to the need for new ethics to meet the challenges of new technology: "When we juxtapose technology and morals, as we must, we should learn to expect that technology will stretch, and often break, the categories for thought that previously defined our moral view."[2] Deane-Drummond brings eschatology and ethics to bear on this challenge: "A fundamental hope for Christian believers is hope in the resurrection. Christianity is also realistic about the possibility of human sin, and the need to tackle attitudes that lead to the breakdown of communities through all forms of injustice and violence."[3] Beginning from here, let us see where this leads.[4]

In this chapter I "Google" a map that tracks the direction in which transhumanists would like to take the human race. The transhumanist destination is a posthuman species characterized by good health, enhanced intelligence, and perhaps even immortality. The road to get there has been paved by the conflation of biological evolution and technological progress. Even though the transhumanist engine is fueled by a blend of genetics, nanotechnology, and robotics (GNR), out of the transhumanist exhaust pipe comes reliance upon Social Darwinism in the form of laissez-faire capitalism, an ecological ethic requiring global cooperation, and a denunciation of atavistic religion. Finally, in conclusion, I would like to show how high-speed transhumanism will need to dodge potholes such as secular anxiety regarding technological dehumanization and how it risks getting detoured by theological assessments of the doctrine of progress, human sinfulness, and God's promise for ultimate transformation.

The Transhumanist Destination: A Posthuman Race

Our Google map shows the transhumanist destination to be an enhanced human future, if not a fully *posthuman* future. Why might we want to go there? Because the current human condition is not good enough. It could be better than it is. Evolution has brought us to where we are. Now, through technology, we can speed up evolutionary change and even direct its development. "Transhumanists view human nature as a work-in-progress, a half-baked beginning that we can learn to remold in desirable ways. Current humanity need not be the endpoint of evolution," claims Nick Bostrom.[5]

This destination will be characterized by the liberation of humanity from its inherited limits. According to the "Transhumanist Declaration" of the World Transhumanist Association, "Humanity will be radically changed by technology in the future. We foresee the feasibility of redesigning the human condition, including such parameters as the inevitability of aging, limitations on human and artificial intellects, unchosen psychology, suffering, and our confinement to the planet earth."[6]

Traveling the evolutionary highway to date has been slow. Now we can accelerate the speed of change. "Transhumanism is the view that humans should (or should be permitted to) use technology to remake human nature," is the definition offered by Heidi Campbell and Mark Walker.[7] It is a science and a philosophy that seeks to employ genetic technology, information technology, and nanotechnology to greatly enhance the healthy life spans of persons, increase intelligence, and make us humans happier and more virtuous. The key is to recontextualize humanity in terms of technology. This leads to a vision of a posthuman future characterized by a merging of humanity with technology as the next stage of our human evolution. Humanity plus (H+) is calling us forward. *Posthuman* refers to who we might become if transhuman efforts achieve their goals.

Transhumanism seeks more than merely new technological gadgets. It seeks to construct a philosophy of life, a total worldview, a grand metanarrative. Transhumanists want to replace both the modern and postmodern narratives. What is wrong with modernism? Our Western religious tradition has failed to hold us together in our modern age. What is wrong with postmodernism? Postmodernism is failing, because this nihilistic philosophy refuses to recognize the gifts of the modern scientific age, namely, reason and progress. What we need at this moment is an inspiring philosophy that reveres scientific reason and that will pull us toward a positive future. To meet this post-post-modern need, transhumanists offer a "totalized philosophical system" with a three-level worldview—metaphysical, psychological level, and ethical.[8]

First comes the metaphysical or cosmological level. Here the transhumanist sees a world in a "process of evolutionary complexification toward ever more complex structures, forms, and operations." Second comes the psychological level. Here transhumanists believe that we human beings are "imbued with the innate Will to Evolve—an instinctive drive to expand abilities in pursuit of ever-increasing survivability and well-being." And third comes the ethical level. Here "we should seek to *foster* our innate Will to Evolve, by continually striving to expand our abilities throughout life. By acting in harmony with the essential nature of the evolutionary process—complexification—we may discover a new sense of purpose, direction, and meaning to life, and come to feel ourselves *at home in the world* once more" (emphasis in the original).[9] What Simon Young plans is to replace "Darwinian Evolution with Designer Evolution—from slavery to the selfish genes to conscious self-rule by the human mind."[10]

Evolution and progress are two ideas that fit together like a gun and a bullet. "That technological progress is generally desirable from a transhumanist point of view is also self-evident,"[11] Bostrom says with a touch of understatement. This technological progress will allegedly shoot the human race like a cannon ball over its previous barriers. "Transhumanism has roots in secular humanist thinking, yet is more radical in that it . . . direct[s] application of medicine and technology to overcome some of our basic biological limits."[12] Young proffers "the belief in overcoming human limitations through reason, science, and technology."[13]

One of the limits to be overcome is death, preceded by the aging process. Death can be overcome in two ways, either through radical life extension or cybernetic immortality. Through advances in GNR, human life can be extended for millennia. Unless befallen by accident, our biological life will continue indefinitely. Aubrey de Grey says that he is "not in favor of aging." When one is not in favor of something, then it is time to apply technology to overcome it. This is what de Grey plans. If we could eliminate aging, then "we will be in possession of indefinite youth. We will die only from the sort of causes that young people die of today—accidents, suicide, homicide, and so on—but not of the age-related diseases that account for the vast majority of deaths in the industrialized world today."[14]

The second transhumanist method for overcoming death is cybernetic immortality. Whereas in the past we have been prisoners of our biology, in the future we will become liberated. Our liberation will come through enhanced intelligence. This enhanced intelligence will be removed from our bodies and placed in computer hardware for a disembodied immortal existence. Posthuman intelligence will find a way to remove itself from our deteriorating bodies and establish a much more secure substrate for endurance. Our mental lives in the future may take place within a computer or on the internet. What we have previously known as *Homo sapiens* will be replaced by *Homo cyberneticus*. "*As humanism freed us from the chains of superstition, let transhumanism free us from our biological chains*" (emphasis in the original).[15]

Once liberated from the limits of aging or even from our physical bodies themselves, the expansion of human intelligence would be limited only by the size of our universe. What Hans Moravec foresees is a cosmic imbuing of matter with consciousness: "Liberated from biological slavery, an immortalized species, *Homo cyberniticus*, will set out for the stars. Conscious life will gradually spread throughout the galaxy . . . until finally, in the unimaginably distant future, the whole universe has come alive, awakened to its own nature—a cosmic mind become conscious of itself as a living entity—omniscient, omnipotent, omnipresent."[16] The entire universe will be converted into an "extended thinking entity."[17]

The proud aggressiveness of the transhumanist reminds us of Prometheus and the promethean spirit. Here is the promethean promise: We humans will arrest from the gods and from nature the principles and resources we need to take our destiny into our own hands. With a wave of the philosophical hand, we will expel the old fatalisms, the naysayers, the

Luddites. "Bio-fatalism will increasingly be replaced by techno-can-do-ism—the belief in the power of the new technology to free us from the limitations of our bodies and minds. . . . In the twenty-first century, the belief in the Fall of Man will be replaced by the belief in his inevitable transcendence—through Superbiology."[18] The torch of Prometheus will lead us into the new world of transhumanism. "Let us cast aside cowardice and seize the torch of Prometheus with both hands."[19]

Such Promethean hubris regarding progress in technology is accompanied by a utopian vision, a vision of future human fulfillment or even post-human fulfillment in a kingdom where rational intelligence has transcended its previous biological imprisonment. Not only as individuals but also as a social community and even as a cosmic community, we will experience ecstatic human flourishing, the abundant life of which previous religious visionaries could only dream. This is where the transhumanists would like to take us.

Crossing the Singularity Bridge to Posthumanity

The road to the enhanced human or the posthuman will need to cross the bridge into higher intelligence, a new level of intelligence that will take over evolutionary advance from that point on. We might label this threshold "the Singularity Bridge." It is a toll bridge. Passage requires paying a toll in the form of granting an assumption: that our mind can be reduced to, and exhausted by, what happens in the brain.

"You are your brain," we hear *Time* magazine telling us.[20] This is a handy assumption because, if it is true, then if we can transform the human brain, we can transform humanity itself. This assumption leads to the on-ramp of the Singularity Bridge—the creation of smarter-than-human intelligence.[21]

The Singularity belongs to the vision of technoprophet Ray Kurzweil. The Singularity is a dramatic future event—not in the distant future but rather just around the corner, in 2045 to be exact.[22] Leading up to the Singularity, we will see how the pace of technological change will be so rapid and its impact so deep that human life will be irreversibly transformed. The nose on this transformation face will be enhanced human intelligence. What follows this nose will be the observation that human intelligence will leap from human bodies to machines, making high-technology machines more human than we are. This can happen because intelligence is not dependent upon our biological substrate; rather, as information in patterns, intelligence can be extricated from our bodies. Our intelligence can live on in an enhanced form even when extricated from our bodies and placed in a computer. As Kurzweil explains, "Uploading a human brain means scanning all of its salient details and then reinstantiating those details into a suitably powerful computational substrate. This process would capture a person's entire personality, memory, skills, and history."[23]

Kurzweil's proposal requires that we accept the dubious idea that human intelligence can be disembodied, separated from the brain, and "uploaded." On the bright side, however, we would have new bodies, namely, machines. "Future machines will be human even if they are not biological," writes Kurzweil. "This will be the next step in evolution."[24] Rather than a biological substrate, humans of a future generation will rely upon a machine substrate. When we have escaped our biological limitations, we will be able to program a much longer life, a disembodied yet intelligent life. "The Singularity will allow us to transcend these limitations of our biological bodies and brains. We will gain power over our fates. Our mortality will be in our own hands. We will be able to live as long as we want. . . . By the end of this century, the nonbiological portion of our intelligence will be trillions of trillions of times more powerful than unaided human intelligence."[25]

Would living in cyberspace seem attractive? Would it be lonely? No. One would not be alone. One's cybermind would be in community with all other cyberminds, a variant on Teilhard's Noosphere. One might even celebrate a new higher level of community. This is what Margaret Wertheim celebrates. Despite the dangers lurking in our computers, she thanks cyberspace for establishing a network of relationships. Further, the global community of electronic relationships is eliciting a sense of responsibility toward one another. "If cyberspace teaches us anything," she writes, "it is that the worlds we conceive . . . are communal projects requiring ongoing communal responsibility."[26] Once Kurzweil has successfully uploaded our minds into cyberspace, we will enjoy a communal network of shared intelligence.

Evolutionary travel has brought us thus far. We have further to go, however, according to the transhumanists. Our generation has the opportunity to enhance our intelligence, to advance still further in evolutionary development. Computers, along with GNR, are all tools whereby we can build a dramatically new future for abundant living and cosmic community.

Let us remind ourselves of the close tie assumed here between biological evolution and technological progress. Kurzweil sees the latter as an extension of the former. The key characteristic of both evolutionary and technological progress is inevitability, according to Kurzweil. Both natural evolution and human technology benefit from a guiding purpose, a built-in purpose. And this built-in logos or entelechy virtually guarantees the future he is forecasting. What is this built-in purpose? Increased intelligence. "The purpose of the universe reflects the same purpose as our lives: to move toward greater intelligence and knowledge. . . . We will within this century be ready to infuse our solar system with our intelligence through self-replicating non-biological intelligence. It will then spread out to the rest of the universe."[27]

The method for getting there from here is this: applying our existing intelligence to leaping the hurdles that currently need technological transcending. "Insight from the brain reverse-engineering effort, overall research in developing AI [artificial intelligence] algorithms, and ongoing exponential gains in computing platforms make strong AI (AI at human levels and beyond) inevitable. Once AI achieves human levels, it will necessarily soar past it because it will combine the strengths of human intelligence with the speed, memory capacity, and knowledge sharing that nonbiological intelligence already exhibits."[28] Note Kurzweil's confident vocabulary—"inevitable" and "necessary." Simon Young makes this explicit: "The furtherance of human evolution through advanced biotechnology is not only possible, but *inevitable*" (emphasis in the original).[29]

Deane-Drummond applies the term *hyperhumanism* to describe transhumanist prometheanism. Hyperhumanism is the questionable assumption or unfounded belief that humanity is in control of its own history and its own evolutionary future. "It would be a mark of intense hubris marked with political overtones of eugenics to expect that humans can control their own evolution."[30] Can technological progress get us there? Deane-Drummond is doubtful.

Even if evolution and progress will take us there, do we really want to get to this place? Before electing to travel this road, one might want to pause to point out that once we get there, it might not be *we ourselves* who have arrived. Those arriving would be our progeny, not us. Should we complain about the loss of our identity when we are replaced by posthumans who transcend us? No, says Bostrom. "We may favor future people being posthuman rather than human, if the posthumans would lead lives more worthwhile than the alternative humans would. Any reasons stemming from such considerations would not depend on the assumption that we ourselves could become posthuman beings."[31] Because our lives today are less "worthwhile," our high-minded and selfless values place us in a position to greet with appreciation our replacement by a race of higher, more intelligent, more perfected beings. This is the transhumanist vision.

The Ethical Exhaust Pipe: Laissez-Faire Capitalism, Ecological Cooperation, and the Denunciation of Religion

To what kind of ethical deliberation or moral code might transhumanism lead? It leads in three directions. One direction is toward laissez-faire capitalism, a contemporary copy of nineteenth-century Social Darwinism.

Why take a position on capitalism? Because only the wealthy sectors of the modern economy are sufficiently flushed with money to afford to invest in GNR. Capital investment and technological advance provide cyclical support for one another. Investors invest in GNR, and the sales earnings from GNR increase the amount of capital available for reinvestment. "It's the economic imperative of a competitive marketplace that is the primary force driving technology forward and fueling the law of accelerating returns. . . . Economic imperative is the equivalent of survival in biological evolution."[32] What we find here is an ethical principle—the Will to Evolve, mentioned above—drawn from evolutionary biology and applied to economics, the "survival of the fittest." Transhumanism is not a philosophy for the losers, for the poor who are slated to be left behind in the struggle for existence.

A second direction taken by transhumanist ethical thinking is toward increased cooperation, even altruism or benevolence. Support for altruism takes the form of a commonsense admonition to cooperate with one other for the betterment of all. Benevolence is more highly valued than selfishness, according to transhumanist ethics. When this direction is taken, the Darwinian struggle for existence with its competitive aggression, is replaced by a liberal ethic. Curiously, we ordinarily think this second direction would take one far away from the Social Darwinism described above.

A third direction denounces religious traditions for being conservative, and thus resistant to the advance of progress. Because religion allegedly roots itself in the ancient past and defends today's status quo with rigid dogma, it puts up stop signs in an attempt to prevent self-modification through technological progress. Whether this is an accurate picture of religion or not, transhumanists believe that if they are to drive the wider society toward their vision of a better future, religious stop signs will need to be removed.

Even though transhumanists invoke the term "evolution" to refer both to humanity's past and to its future progress, these two differ. Evolution's past was characterized by the struggle for existence, the survival of the fittest. Evolution's future, in contrast, appears to be concerned with human fulfillment. The provolutionist Jürgen Moltmann ponders this. If in our era of biomedical progress, human existence is no longer oriented toward mere survival, then we are ready to reorient our lives around a new purpose: fulfillment. Darwinian values that may have supported the survival of the fittest will need replacing by values that promote cooperation and social harmony. "The change in human interests evoked by biomedical progress can be described as a transition from the struggle for existence to striving for fulfillment," writes Moltmann. "The principle of self-preservation against others can be transformed into the principle of self-fulfillment in the other. Systems of aggression can be overcome by systems of co-operation."[33]

The implication for transhumanist ethics is this: despite the conflation of biological evolution and technological progress, Darwinian values such as self-preservation in the competition for existence cannot be thought to be progressive in light of the picture of the future that the transhumanists are painting. Yet their reliance upon the Will to Evolve in the form of laissez-faire capitalism reiterates the nineteenth-century reliance on Social Darwinism, the very value system that apparently needs replacing. In sum, transhumanist ethics is torn by a tension between the capitalist values adhering to the survival-of-the-fittest principle and the altruistic values of a benevolent community.

The Transhumanist Denunciation of Religion

Transhumanists denounce religion. Why? Because what they think they see in front of them are roadblocks put there by religion. Religion, they believe, is Luddite. Through the eyes of today's transhumanists, religion looks like a roadblock, an obstruction.

Simon Young provides an example of one who would like to clear religious blockage to make way for transhumanism. He assumes that a religious faith in God is necessarily atavistic and recalcitrant. After all, if God created the world the way it is, then it follows that it is immoral to change it. If God allowed a child to be born with a genetic defect, it follows that it is immoral for medical therapists to repair it. This is Young's logic, applicable to the Christian faith if not other religions: "The greatest threat to humanity's continuing evolution is theistic opposition to Superbiology in the name of a belief system based on blind faith in the absence of evidence."[34]

What the transhumanists think they see in religion is an atavistic commitment to the past, to the status quo, to resistance against anything new. This image is misleading, although I must admit that some religious reactions to scientific and technological advances can take Luddite form. Be that as it may, Christian theology strongly affirms change. This religious tradition even looks forward to radical transformation and, in anticipation, provolutionary creativity. The reluctance to embrace progress on the part of theologians does not come from a posture of resistance to change. Rather, it comes from an entirely different source: a critique of the naïveté on the part of those who put their faith in progress, especially technological progress. Deane-Drummond makes this clear: "We need not totally reject . . . technology, but appreciate its proper limits according to particular goals that express the common good."[35]

What about the transhumanist attempt to attain everlasting life? Out of an apparent fear that religious tradition might attempt to slow down technological innovation, transhumanists accuse religious representatives of holding a vested interest in provenance over matters of death and immortality. One of the impediments to the advance toward cybernetic immortality is religion, they say. Religion stands in the way. Religion threatens to block progress. This is because religion has traditionally sought to provide a palliative for people faced with death. Religion brings an acceptance of death, and comfort with that acceptance. Therefore Kurzweil—ready in Promethean style to engage in combat with traditional religion—wants to defy death and use nanotechnology as a weapon to defeat death. He explains: "The primary role of traditional religion is deathist rationalization—that is, rationalizing the tragedy of death as a good thing."[36] To benefit from what the Singularity can bring, we need to overcome our "deathist" rationalization. We need to sweep traditional religion out of our road.

Given what was mentioned just above, it would appear to me that any improvement in human health or even longevity would be greeted by Christian provolutionists as a blessing from science, a gift for which to be thankful. No theological recalcitrance would block progress toward human betterment through medical technology. Conversely, a Christian theologian is likely to contend that neither the extension of the present life span nor cybernetic immortality corresponds to the biblical vision of resurrection from the dead. "The immortality promised by the likes of Kurzweil . . . remains a very limited one and falls far short of the Christian hope and expectation of redemption," writes Gregory Peterson.[37] Our redemption through resurrection into the new creation does not correspond to physical longevity or cybernetic immortality.

Brent Waters treats posthumanists as if they offer a worldview comparable to, though partially differing from, the Christian worldview. Both posthumanists and Christians

agree that humans need to be released from their current plight. For posthumanists, this is achieved through technologically driven transformation, while Christians believe they are transformed by their life in Christ. Both agree that death is the final enemy. One conquers this foe by extending longevity and perhaps achieving virtual immortality, while the other is resurrected into the eternal life of God. Consequently, both place their hope in a future that at present appears as little more than a puzzling reflection in a mirror: One can only speculate what life will be like in a posthuman world, or a new Heaven and Earth.[38]

Two Roads to the Future: Futurology and Eschatology

Theologians work with two distinctive yet complementary ways for viewing the future. The first way is to foresee the future as growth, as an actualization of potentials residing in the present or past. The second way is to
anticipate something new, to prophesy a coming new reality. The first can
be identified with the Latin term *futurum*, which suggests growth, development, maturation, or fruition. An oak tree is the actualized *futurum* of a
potential that already exists in the acorn. The Latin term *adventus*, in contrast, is the appearance of something new—a first, so to speak. It is an eschatological future that can be expected or hoped for, but it cannot be planned
for. Whereas *futurum* provides an image of the future that can result from
present trends, *adventus* provides a vision of a future that only God can make
happen.[39]

Futurists or futurologists project scenarios based upon *futurum*. Theologians try to draw out the implications of God's promise for *adventus*. The
Roman Catholic theologian Karl Rahner spoke of God's future as a "mystery," as a coming reality beyond our rational control. Human consciousness
transcends present reality with an openness toward the future, to be sure,
Rahner said; but we must rely on the fact that "this future wills to give itself
through its own self-communication, . . . which is still in the process of historical realization."[40] The Lutheran theologian Carl Braaten sharply defined
the difference between futurology and eschatology: "A crucial difference
between secular futurology and Christian eschatology is this: The future in
secular futurology is *reached* by a process of the world's *becoming*. The future
in Christian eschatology *arrives* by the *coming* of God's kingdom. The one is
a *becoming* and the other a *coming*."[41]

In light of these two understandings of the future, it is clear that the concept with which transhumanists work is the future as *futurum*, the future as a
futurologist would grasp it.[42] New and startling things await us in the future,
but the way from here to there is growth, technological advance. Human
and posthuman flourishing will be the result of step-by-step advances. This
understanding of the posthuman future depends on a related concept: progress.[43] Before we turn to the zealous transhumanist faith in progress, let us
point out a pothole, namely, anxiety about dehumanization. A fear that technology is already dehumanizing us has colored our vision since the Industrial Revolution, and the transhumanist forecast that we humans will become
extinct in favor of a posthumanist species will only exacerbate this anxiety.

Anxiety about Dehumanization

In the wake of World War II philosophers-cum-futurists such as Georgetown University's Victor Ferkiss have wrestled with the role of technology in bearing our civilization toward its future. Not merely the machines we invent are relevant. Perhaps more relevant is the technological mindset, the cultural incorporation of the machine into our self-understanding as human beings. The nearly primordial concept of *techne* or *technique* refers to the complex of standardized means for attaining a predetermined result. The technical mind converts otherwise spontaneous and unreflective behavior into behavior that is deliberate and rationalized. What distinguishes our modern world is the sheer delight we take in *technique*, finding fascination at more complex computers, faster jets, and bigger bombs. New nouns such as "technological man" or "technological civilization" have come to describe the ever-expanding and apparently irreversible rule of technique in all domains of life. Technique has not only expanded our practical lives; it has also entered into our inner lives. Technique has become constitutive of the identity of modern human being. "Technology is what has made man man," wrote Ferkiss.[44]

The "technological man" of the late 1960s looks much like the techno-sapien heralded by today's transhumanists. Now, we might ask: Could progress take us to the point where a fully "technological man," or perhaps a fully "technologized humanity," could emerge? To believe that such a thing is possible, let alone desirable, is to embrace a myth. "Technological man is more myth than reality," warned Ferkiss.[45] Why? Because of the split between technique and value. Technique is still pressed into the service of values that transcend it, whether we observe this or not. And what critical observers have seen during the industrial age in the modern West is the subordination of both science and technology into the service of economic greed and political domination. Today's technology is still supported and guided by yesterday's bourgeois values. Nothing suggests that this arrangement will change. As Ferkiss observes, "What if the new man combines the animal irrationality of primitive man with the calculated greed and power-lust of industrial man, while possessing the virtually Godlike powers granted him by technology? This would be the ultimate horror."[46]

This older literature is quite relevant to our analysis of the transhumanist project. Note two things. First, transhumanism masquerades as value-free science responding to what nature tells us; yet this very divestment of traditional religious values is susceptible to bourgeois financial interests. Second, note how transhumanists believe in an inherent alliance between transhumanist progress and free market capitalism. The values allegedly inherent within evolution and progress will not be able to sustain themselves in the face of the pressure to serve the demands of the funders. Money talks. What money says goes. No escape exists to liberate technological progress from the vested interests of the economic and political powers that make such progress possible. Despite their feeble whisperings of liberal values such as altruism, cooperation, and ecology, the progress transhumanists anticipate will be unavoidably diverted into the service of consolidating and expanding the wealth of its investors.

More Anxiety about Dehumanization

Among the critics of the transhumanist movement, we find the historian Francis Fukuyama. He fears that self-modification will threaten what evolution has already bequeathed to the human race—its dignity: "We want to protect the full range of our complex, evolved natures against attempts at self-modification. We do not want to disrupt either the unity or the continuity of human nature, and thereby the human rights that are based on it."[47] Our natural history has provided the human race with foundations for dignity, rights, and civilization. To change this foundation risks a loss of these qualities. Curiously, Fukuyama accepts the past changes in biology wrought by evolution while opposing future changes to be brought by technology. What is important for our analysis here, however, is the anxiety awakened by transhumanism about the possible loss of human identity and dignity.

Dehumanization comes in two forms: first, the subordination of human values to impersonal technological advance; and, second, the anticipation that humanity will become extinct when the posthuman species evolves. Bill Joy confronted us with the second form vividly in his landmark essay "Why the Future Doesn't Need Us." Can we imagine a future in which we, the members of the human race as we know it, will be no longer? Will downloading our intelligence into a machine threaten the continuation of our humanity? "But if we are downloaded into our technology," Joy asks, "what are the chances that we will thereafter be ourselves or even human?"[48] The transformation of the natural world around us, along with the transformation of ourselves into something new that surpasses us, raises a question: Will the kind of technological progress advocated by the transhumanists actually dehumanize us? Would such a dehumanization be due to this specific technological proposal, or would it be due to the very nature of the technique itself?

Watching the incorporation of technique into human self-understanding has alarmed both theologians and secular humanists for a half century now. Some fear that technology applied to the inner life dehumanizes us, that it cuts us off from our otherwise spontaneous joy at being natural creatures. "Technique is opposed to nature," writes the French social critic and Reformed theologian Jacques Ellul. "It destroys, eliminates, or subordinates the natural world, and does not allow this world to restore itself or even to enter into a symbiotic relation with it."[49] Now Ellul's pitting human nature in opposition to technique is a bit extreme, because most anthropologies would affirm that the pursuit of technological innovation is one of the obvious attributes of human nature. We are *Homo faber*, the species that makes things. So the threat of dehumanization comes not from technological advance per se; rather, the threat comes from our temptation to so identify with our technological production that we forget our relationship to the natural world. To protect us from such forgetfulness, Ferkiss proposes a new norm: "Man is part of nature and therefore cannot be its conqueror and indeed he owes it some respect."[50] A theological humanist, Lund University's Ulf Görman, even includes mortality in the definition of what constitutes our humanness: "I would like to argue that these everlasting immortals are not humans in the full sense of our understanding . . . because they lack an important existential dimension of human life."[51] In sum, the advance to *the posthuman* repulses those who appreciate what we have come to know as *the human*.

Just how it is that technology threatens our humanity is subtle. On the one hand, the transhumanists propose a technology that will enhance our humanity, or at least the intelligent aspect of humanity. On the other hand, once technology takes over and replicates itself, it will leave our present stage of humanity in the evolutionary dust. An emerging posthumanity will replace us. We might ask: If we replace ourselves with posthumanity, will we have given expression to our essential human potential for self-transcendence through technology? Just how should we think about this?

If yesterday's futurists could speak to today's challenge, they would most likely warn us of tendencies within us to surrender what is human to the mindset of technique. Ferkiss said: "While it is untrue that technology determines the future independently of human volition, there is no question that that human individuals and human society are increasingly under pressure to conform to the demands of technological efficiency, and there is a real possibility that the essence of humanity will be lost in the process, that human history will come to an end and be converted into a mere prelude to the history of a posthuman society in which machines rather than men rule."[52] But Ferkiss admonishes us to avoid this pitfall: "Man must maintain the distinction between himself and the machines of his creation. . . . Not only must man stand above the machine, he must be in control of his own evolution."[53] Almost presciently anticipating today's proposal to create a posthuman intelligence, Ferkiss declares that we should preserve our humanness;

we should maintain today's humanity over against the temptation to replace it with something more advanced: "Man's greatest need is not to transcend his species as such but to develop it fully. . . . Man is not a superape; he is no longer an ape at all. Before we abandon man for a machine-man or a genetic mutant, we should learn what he can do in his present form once liberated from hunger, fear and ignorance."[54] Perhaps Ferkiss the humanist would represent the religious roadblock the transhumanists would like to clear out of the way.

Now this observation that we human beings belong to nature and are embedded in nature is important, to be sure; yet this is not the point I would like to stress here. What is more important to the present analysis is the naive sense of control or false sense of dominance that technological victories over nature might elicit. The University of Chicago theologian David Tracy alerts us to the dangers of sacrificing our better judgment to naive trust in technological progress: "Now *techne* becomes the product of the will to domination, power and control, . . . a power on its own, leveling all culture; annihilating all at-home-ness in the cosmos, uprooting all other questions in favor of those questions under its control; producing a planetary thought-world where instrumental reason, and it alone, will pass as thought. . . . The object cannot think. The subject will not. We began as technical agents of our willful destiny. We seem to end as technicized spectators at our own execution."[55]

A Theological Critique of Progress

As pointed out above, the transhumanists place their faith and trust in a combination of biological evolution and technological progress. In fact, these two are conflated. Or rather, biological evolution is incorporated within the more comprehensive doctrine of progress. Is this transhumanist belief acceptable to contemporary science? Perhaps not. Many leading evolutionary theorists—including Ernst Mayr, Stephen Jay Gould, and Francisco Ayala—refute the notion that progress is built into the process of evolutionary change. But it is not my agenda here to defend this scientific position. Instead, I would like to turn to distinctively theological resources to assess the doctrine of progress, asking if *futurum* alone can realistically deliver all that transhumanists promise.

Reinhold Niebuhr and his followers provide appropriate theological resources for addressing the doctrine of progress. In the tradition of Augustine and Martin Luther, they proffered a version of "Christian realism" regarding the sinful condition in which we human beings find ourselves; and they cautioned against overestimating what we can achieve within history apart from the gracious action of God.

Already in his pre–World War II writings, Niebuhr shows awareness that our modern post-Enlightenment culture, which plays host to both natural science and European imperialism, is a branch growing on a larger historical tree. The tree's trunk stands with roots in classical Greece and Rome as well as in the soil of Israel's history and the Christian Bible. The modern idea of progress, he avers, is both an outgrowth and a pruned version of biblical eschatology. The prophets and the apocalypticists of Scripture saw human history as dynamic, as changing, as moving from promise to fulfillment. But human advance is also subject to divine judgment. What this means is that all events within history are ambiguous—that is, the advance of each human potential can lead to either a good actualization or an evil actualization. Unambiguous goodness is not guaranteed by progress. Only eschatologically—only at the advent of God's Kingdom, which will come by an act of divine grace—will unambiguous fulfillment be possible. In the meantime, we live in the paradox of being able to envision fulfillment while experiencing the inescapable dialectic of success and failure.

For Niebuhr, progress and modern culture belong together like cheese and crackers: "The idea of progress is the underlying presupposition of what may be broadly defined as 'liberal' culture. If that assumption is challenged the whole structure of meaning in the liberal world is imperiled. . . . The creed is nevertheless highly dubious. . . . It is false in so far as all historical processes are ambiguous."[56] The ambiguity of which Niebuhr speaks is the ever-present potential created by human freedom, namely, the potential to choose evil and chaos along with what is good and fulfilling.

The problem is that today's believers in progress are blind to this ambiguity. They trust that inherent to the progress of history is a built-in *telos*, or guiding principle, that transforms otherwise meaningless growth into a process of betterment. This belief is a truncation of the biblical eschatology that preceded it. It is an outgrowth of the effect of Scripture on Western culture, to be sure; but the concept of progress prunes off this growth the previous recognition of the ineluctable continuation of creative evil. "The 'idea of progress,' the most characteristic and firmly held article in the credo of modern man, is the inevitable philosophy of history emerging from the Renaissance. This result was achieved by combining the classical confidence in man with the Biblical confidence in the meaningfulness of history. It must be observed, however, that history is given a simpler meaning than that envisaged in the prophetic-Biblical view. . . . [Progress] did not recognize that history is filled with endless possibilities *of good and evil.* . . . It did not recognize that every new human potency may be an instrument of chaos as well as of order; and that history, therefore, has no solution of its own problem" (emphasis in the original).[57]

The Computer Virus and Sin

At this point I cannot avoid introducing the phenomenon of the computer virus. In the case of the computer virus, we find an example of a nonbiological self-replicating entity that has appeared on the scene along with the spread of Internet communication. This software pathogen threatens to destroy our computer network medium. What is Kurzweil's interpretation? "Although software pathogens remain a concern, the danger exists mostly at a nuisance level," he comments. Then he adds: "When we have software running in our brains and bodies and controlling the world's nanobot immune system, the stakes will be immeasurably greater."[58]

In light of what Niebuhr has said, I recommend that we pause for a moment to consider the significance of the computer virus for understanding the human condition. The invention of the computer virus is an invention with one sole purpose: to destroy. Despite the benefits or even blessings of computer connections around the world, something at work in the human mind leads to the development of brute and unmitigated destruction. No increase in human intelligence or advance in technology will alter this ever-lurking human proclivity.

A sweeping technological optimism tends to dismiss awareness of this human weakness. But if we are to be realistic, we require an accurate portrayal of the human situation. It requires an honest recognition of human sinfulness. At any time and in any place, otherwise happy and fulfilled human beings may initiate evil and destruction. This ever-present risk of sinful activity is a universal contingent—that is, though unnecessary, it is always and everywhere possible. "Sin is natural for man in the sense that it is universal but not in the sense that it is necessary."[59] At the birth of the computer age, we should have been able to predict the coming of the computer virus, or something like it. Now, at the birth of transhumanist technology, similar predictions would be in order. A transhumanist spirituality would need to incorporate this kind of realism regarding human nature, a human nature not capable of changing through the augmentation of intelligence.

Human Progress under Divine Judgment

The pothole in the transhumanist road that Christian theologians point out is the naïveté with which believers in progress remove the ambiguities of human history, which leads them to maintain confidence in the good that progress can bring while denying the potential growth of evil. What the theologian ought to steadfastly maintain is that our vision of human abundance and flowering must hold on to its transcendence; we must hold on to the judgment that the eschatological Kingdom of God renders against the accomplishments of human history. "There is a great temptation today to confuse sociological evolution with spiritual progress," writes Ellul. "The Bible expressly tells us that the history of mankind ends in judgment."[60]

What is the antidote to transhumanist naïvete? It is provolutionary creativity combined with reliance upon a transcendent judgment against human history. A cursory review of modern history calls out for such divine judgment. The theologian Paul Jersild points a cautious way: "In some respects, a more civilized society does emerge with the evolution of cultures, but there is ample evidence that evolving societies invent still more horrific ways to exalt themselves and destroy their neighbors. Evolution, whether biological or cultural, does not mean inexorable progress on the road toward perfection."[61] In sum, we should move forward, but we should not presume that progress in every respect is inevitable or guaranteed. Technological advance does not belong to an underlying or inevitable advance in human goodness or human achievement.

A Provolutionary Conclusion

Perhaps my conclusion is now obvious. It appears to me that members of the transhumanist school of thought are naive about human nature and that they are overestimating what they can accomplish through technological innovation. They are naive because they take insufficient account of the human propensity for using neutral or even good things for selfish purposes, which results in chaos and suffering. The assumption that the transhumanists seem to make that both biological evolution and technological progress have their own built-in entelechy or purpose from which we can derive our social ethic overlooks the threat to their values posed by the funders. By depending on private capital and even building laissez-faire capitalism into their value system, they risk subjugating all their technological achievements to the values of the bourgeois class. The result will be technological advances that benefit these investors to the detriment of the wider society and the ecosphere they would like to rehabilitate.

The transhumanist forecast of a future replete with cybernetic immortality and cosmic consciousness seems extravagant and fantastic. Whether it is possible for our intelligence and self-consciousness to be reduced to information patterns and then uploaded on to a nonbiological substrate is not a question I can address here. But I would like to point out that there is no warrant for believing that all our human problems will be solved by transhumanist technology. There is no warrant for thinking that the currently selfish human race will be able to transform itself into an altruistic or benevolent one. There is no warrant for thinking that we human beings with our history of economic injustice and ecologically unhealthy habits are willing or able, on our own, to eliminate poverty and protect the ecosphere. No amount of increased intelligence will redeem us from what the theologians call *sin*.

In previous works dealing with futurology, I have called this the *eschatological problem*. I ask: How do we get there from here? If we in the human race have been responsible for selfishness, economic injustice, and environmental degradation, how can we then become capable of benevolence, economic justice, and ecological health? How can a leopard change its spots? What transhumanists are hoping for is *adventus*, but they have only *futurum* to work with. A realistic element of provolutionary thinking is the expectation and hope for eschatological transformation.

What is important to the theologian is God's promise that some of what appears in the transhumanist vision will come to pass. But the transformation of the human heart so that it exudes benevolence and justice will require more than *futurum* can deliver. It will require divine grace, what only *adventus* can accomplish. The advent of the new creation will require much more than what our evolutionary history by itself can deliver. It will require God's transforming power. Increased human intelligence cannot on its own accomplish what it will take divine grace to make happen.

In sum, a Christian theologian can only encourage continued scientific research into genetics and nanotechnology when the goals are improved human health and well-being. Attempts to enhance human intelligence through technological augmentation might also be greeted with approval, although probably not with overwhelming enthusiasm. Because the theologian looks forward to the advent of divine transformation, he or she can celebrate anticipatory transformations brought about by advances in science and technology. Provolutionary theology need not be recalcitrant or Luddite. Provolutionary theology can be ready to celebrate technological breakthroughs while remaining realistic about what to expect from human nature.

Notes

1. Moltmann, *Religion, Revolution, and the Future*, 32.
2. Cole-Turner, "Religion Meets Research," 11.
3. Deane-Drummond, "Future Perfect?" 182.

4. My analysis here extends that of earlier studies: Peters, "Perfect Humans"; Peters, "Transhumanism"; and Peters, *Anticipating Omega*, esp. the two chapters on the posthuman soul.

5. Bostrom, "Transhumanist Values."

6. World Transhumanist Association, "Transhumanist Declaration." Transhumanism is an expansion on *extropianism*. Extropy, in contrast to entropy, refers to a system's capacity for growth based upon its functional order, intelligence, vitality, energy, and experience. Extropianism or extropism is a set of values oriented toward improving the human condition through technology that might someday bring immortality.

7. Campbell and Walker, "Religion and Transhumanism," 1.

8. Young, *Designer Evolution*, 87.

9. Ibid., 19; also see 202.

10. Ibid., 207.

11. Bostrom, "Transhumanist Values."

12. Ibid.

13. Kurzweil, *Singularity*, 15.

14. de Grey, "Foreword: Forever Young," 9.

15. Young, *Designer Evolution*, 32.

16. Moravec, *Mind Children*, 44.

17. Ibid., 116.

18. Young, *Designer Evolution*, 20.

19. Ibid., 40.

20. Kluger, "New Map of the Brain."

21. The Singularitarians are friends of the Singularity, believers who are working to make it happen. E.g., the Singularity Institute for Artificial Intelligence (www .singinst.org) was founded in 2000 to develop safe artificial intelligence and to raise awareness of both the dangers and potential benefits it believes that artificial intelligence presents.

22. Kurzweil, *Singularity*, 136.

23. Ibid., 198–99.

24. Ibid., 30.

25. Ibid., 9.

26. Wertheim, *Pearly Gates*, 304.

27. Kurzweil, *Singularity*, 372.

28. Ibid., 407.

29. Young, *Designer Evolution*, 22.

30. Deane-Drummond, *Christ and Evolution*, 285.

31. Bostrom, "Transhumanist Values."

32. Kurzweil, *Singularity*, 96.

33. Moltmann, *Future of Creation*, 147.

34. Young, *Designer Evolution*, 324.

35. Deane-Drummond, *Christ and Evolution*, 285.

36. Kurzweil, *Singularity*, 372.

37. Peterson, *Minding God*, 219.

38. Waters, "Saving Us from Ourselves," 190.

39. "*Futurum* means what will be; *adventus* means what is coming." Moltmann, *Coming of God*, 25.

40. Rahner, *Foundations of Christian Faith*, 458.

41. Braaten, *Future of God*, 29.

42. It is my judgment that Robert M. Geraci is mistaken when he insists that the AI movement is apocalyptic (*adventus*) in "Apocalyptic AI." Geraci rightly recognizes that the transhumanists replace divine action with evolutionary progress (p. 159); but then he fails to acknowledge that this implies a nonapocalyptic form of transformation. In addition, he offers a reductionistic interpretation of Jewish and Christian apocalyptic, presuming it is caused by a "breakdown of a proper social order" and a sense of alienation (pp. 140–41, 146–47). He even describes Hans Moravec and Ray Kurzweil as alienated. It is difficult to see how millionaire industrial leaders or authors who publish with Harvard University Press belong to the class of alienated victims of social breakdown.

43. The doctrine of progress and the science of futurology may look different from eschatology, but they are all children of the same religious family. "Alone among the major world religions, and in special contrast to those of the East, Christianity postulated that the world was going somewhere, that the future was not simply an unchanging or cyclically repeating replica of the past. The idea of progress—central to the development of science and the modern world—had its roots in Christian eschatology." Ferkiss, *Technological Man*, 43.

44. Ibid., 36.

45. Ibid., 202.

46. Ibid., 34.

47. Fukuyama, *Our Posthuman Future*, 173.

48. Joy, "Why the Future Doesn't Need Us."

49. Ellul, *Technological Society*, 179.

50. Ferkiss, *Technological Man*, 209.

51. Görman, "Never Too Late," 154.

52. Ferkiss, *Future of Technological Civilization*, 5.

53. Ferkiss, *Technological Man*, 210.

54. Ibid., 216.

55. Tracy, *Analogical Imagination*, 352.

56. Niebuhr, *Nature and Destiny of Man*, vol. 2, 240.

57. Ibid., vol. 2, 154–55.

58. Ibid., 414.

59. Ibid., vol. 1, 242. Robert John Russell introduces the term "universal contingent" in reference to Niebuhr's position. Like human history, nature is also ambiguous—that is, a mixture of beauty and suffering. Russell, "Groaning of Creation."

60. Ellul, *False Presence*, 20.

61. Jersild, "Rethinking the Human Being," 42.

References

Bostrom, Nick. "Transhumanist Values." www.nickbostrom.com/ethics/values.html.

Braaten, Carl E. *The Future of God*. New York: Harper & Row, 1969.

Campbell, Heidi, and Mark Walker. "Religion and Transhumanism: Introducing a Conversation." *Journal of Evolution and Technology* 14, no. 2 (August 2005): 1.

Cole-Turner, Ronald. "Religion Meets Research." In *God and the Embryo: Religious Voices on Stem Cells and Cloning*, edited by Brent Waters and Ronald Cole-Turner. Washington, DC: Georgetown University Press, 2003.

Deane-Drummond, Celia. *Christ and Evolution*. Minneapolis: Fortress Press, 2009.

———. "Future Perfect? God, the Transhuman Future and the Quest for Immortality." In *Future Perfect? God, Medicine and Human Identity*, edited by Celia Deane-Drummond and Peter Manley Scott. London: T. & T. Clark International, 2006.

de Grey, Aubrey. "Foreword: Forever Young." In *Religion and the Implications of Radical Life Extension*, edited by Derek Maher and Calvin Mercer. New York: Palgrave Macmillan, 2010.

Ellul, Jacques. *False Presence of the Kingdom,* translated by C. Edward Hopkin. New York: Seabury Press, 1972.

———. *The Technological Society,* translated by Robert K. Merton. New York: Vintage Books, 1964.

Ferkiss, Victor C. *The Future of Technological Civilization*. New York: George Braziller, 1974.

———. *Technological Man: The Myth and the Reality*. New York: Mentor Books, 1969.

Fukuyama, Francis. *Our Posthuman Future: Consequences of the Biotechnology Revolution*. New York: Farrar, Straus & Giroux, 2002.

Geraci, Robert M. "Apocalyptic AI: Religion and the Promise of Artificial Intelligence." *Journal of the American Academy of Religion* 76, no. 1 (March 2008): 138–66.

Görman, Ulf. "Never Too Late to Live a Little Longer? The Quest for Extended Life and Immortality—Some Ethical Considerations." In *Future Perfect? God, Medicine and Human Identity*, edited by Celia Deane-Drummond and Peter Manley Scott. London: T. & T. Clark International, 2006.

Jersild, Paul. "Rethinking the Human Being in Light of Evolutionary Biology." *Dialog* 47, no. 1 (Spring 2008): 42.

Joy, Bill. "Why the Future Doesn't Need Us." *Wired*, April 2000. www.wired.com/wired/archive/8.04/joy.html .

Kluger, Jeffrey. "The New Map of the Brain." *Time*, January 29, 2007, 57.

Kurzweil, Ray. *The Singularity Is Near: When Humans Transcend Biology*. New York: Penguin, 2005.

Moltmann, Jürgen. *The Coming of God: Christian Eschatology*, translated by Margaret Kohl. Minneapolis: Fortress Press, 1996.

———. *The Future of Creation*, translated by Margaret Kohl. Minneapolis: Fortress Press, 1979.

―――. *Religion, Revolution, and the Future*, translated by Douglas Meeks. New York: Charles Scribner's Sons, 1969.

Moravec, Hans. *Mind Children: The Future of Robot and Human Intelligence*. Cambridge, MA: Harvard University Press, 1988.

Niebuhr, Reinhold. *The Nature and Destiny of Man*. 2 vols. New York: Charles Scribner's Sons, 1941–42.

Peters, Ted. *Anticipating Omega*. Göttingen: Vandenhoeck & Ruprecht, 2007.

―――. "Perfect Humans or Transhumans? In *Future Perfect? God, Medicine and Human Identity*, edited by Celia Deane-Drummond and Peter Manley Scott. London: T. & T. Clark International, 2006.

―――. "Transhumanism and the Post-Human Future: Will Technological Progress Get Us There?" *Global Spiral* 9, no. 3 (June 2008): www.metanexus.net/magazine/tabid/68/id/10546/Default.aspx.

Peterson, Gregory R. *Minding God: Theology and the Cognitive Sciences*. Minneapolis: Fortress Press, 2003.

Rahner, Karl. *Foundations of Christian Faith: An Introduction to the Idea of Christianity*, translated by William V. Dych. New York: Seabury Crossroads Press, 1978.

Russell, Robert John. "The Groaning of Creation: Does God Suffer with All Life?" in *The Evolution of Evil*, edited by Gaymon Bennett, Martinez Hewlett, Ted Peters, and Robert John Russell. Göttingen: Vandenhoeck & Ruprecht, 2008.

Tracy, David. *The Analogical Imagination: Christian Theology and the Culture of Pluralism*. New York: Crossroad, 1981.

Waters, Brent. "Saving Us from Ourselves: Christology, Anthropology and the Seduction of Posthuman Medicine." In *Future Perfect? God, Medicine and Human Identity*, edited by Celia Deane-Drummond and Peter Manley Scott. London: T. & T. Clark International, 2006.

Wertheim, Margaret. *The Pearly Gates of Cyberspace: A History of Space from Dante to the Internet*. New York: W. W. Norton, 1999.

World Transhumanist Association. "Transhumanist Declaration." www.transhumanism.org/index.php/WTA/declaration/.

Young, Simon. *Designer Evolution: A Transhumanist Manifesto*. Amherst, NY: Prometheus Books, 2006.

Chapter Six

The Hopeful Cyborg

STEPHEN GARNER

The transhumanist vision is an end product of the belief that the human condition can be improved through reason, science, and technology. It focuses predominantly upon the autonomous individual, asserting the primacy of reason as a force for personal and therefore societal transformation. Through the use of applied reason, transhumanism asserts that values such as rational thinking, freedom, tolerance, and concern for others are increased, which ultimately leads to an ever-increasing improvement of the human condition.[1] In this way transhumanism claims to offer the hope of a better world.

And yet this proposed vision of a better world is often met with, if not outright hostility, then certainly significant anxiety. In part this anxiety is derived from the way in which transhumanism and other technologically optimistic narratives express their future trajectories through metaphors such as the cyborg. The technologies that transhumanists see converging—nanotechnology, biotechnology, and information technology—reshape and blur not just the traditional essence of what is considered natural but also the concepts used by individuals and communities to understand themselves and the world around them. For example, Jason Scott Robert and Françoise Baylis, who assess proposals to create mixed-species chimeras, argue that "the creation of novel beings that are part human and part nonhuman animal is sufficiently threatening to the social order that for many this is sufficient reason to prohibit any crossing of species boundaries involving human beings."[2] Understandably, this can lead to profoundly unsettling anticipation about the future.

In contemporary Western technoculture one does not have to look very far to see the figure of the cyborg portrayed in popular culture and reflected upon in academia. Popular culture, through media such as film and television, portrays the cyborg figure as the literal fusion of the biological human being with technology, often to the detriment of human identity and dignity. In the academic world the cyborg represents a metaphor for exploring contemporary technoculture, existing as a hybrid figure forming a place where existing categories used to organize the world collapse and restructure themselves. In both cases the cyborg inhabits a newly constructed world that exists in the borderlands of more familiar cultural and experiential terrain.

The cyborg is a generator of "narratives of apprehension" about technology and human technological proclivity. It stands in contrast to many of the traditional ways in which the world is ordered, a disconcerting form that raises questions about human nature, human identity, the relationship between the human and nonhuman in the world, and in particular, how to live wisely and wholesomely in a world constantly being reshaped by technology. As such, the cyborg encourages stories that capture both the anxiety engendered by the perceived negative effects of technology and a sense of wonder and awe at the power and scope of human technological agency.[3]

This is particularly true of questions that are concerned with the very essence of human personhood, about human nature, and the character of the relationship between human beings and the natural world. In commenting on public resistance and antipathy toward particular forms of biotechnology in Britain and Europe at the end of the 1990s, Celia Deane-Drummond and her colleagues write, "It seems conceivable that the intensity of current controversies around genetically modified crops and foods arises in part from the fact that, in their regulation in the public domain, *conflicting ontologies of the person* are making themselves felt in the politics of everyday life" (emphasis added).[4] Ultimately, the questions raised concern not only different ways people describe being human and challenges to a perceived natural order but also how to live wisely and well in a technological world, and especially how to live hopefully.

Cyborgs and Technology as Environment

The term "cyborg" (or "cybernetic organism"), which was coined by Manfred Clynes and Nathan Kline in the 1960s, was part of a proposal to use technology to augment human beings (e.g., astronauts) to survive in harsh environments.[5] The biological cyborg describes an organism, typically human, that has had technological artifacts added to its physical being. Some technological implants—such as synthetic hip replacements, pacemakers, and heart valves—are now taken almost for granted, as are a variety of reproductive technologies. Other technologies, such as prosthetics, continue to advance, along with medical and biotechnologies such as gene therapy, digital implants, cloning, transgenics, xenotransplantation, and pharmaceutical developments.

However, this biological interpretation of the cyborg has less impact than understanding it as a cultural or functional interpretation. For example, the cognitive scientist Andy Clark asserts that human beings are "natural-born cyborgs," in that they have an inherent inclination to form relationships with technologies that expand the human mind outside the limitations of the physical body. In effect, the mind "leaks" into the technological tools and prostheses that human beings use in everyday life. According to Clark, "For we shall be cyborgs not in the merely superficial sense of combining flesh and wires but in the more profound sense of being human-technology symbionts: thinking and reasoning systems whose minds and selves are spread across biological brain and nonbiological circuitry."[6] He argues that it is a mistake to envisage that the most profound and intimate mergers of technology and the human being involve bodily penetration and, at times, replacement. Prostheses, neural implants, and enhanced perceptual and intellectual systems are the norm for the science fiction cyborg, but the impact of everyday appliances and devices such as cellphones and wristwatches is a more significant shaper of human identity and behavior.[7]

Similarly, Donna Haraway argues that all people within a technological society are cyborgs. They may not have technology physically embedded within them, but the boundaries between organism and machine are constantly crossed in everyday social interplay and existence. Technology shapes every aspect of human life, and human identity becomes fluid, because it is forever being shaped by technocultural forces, and thus one cannot be cut off from their influence.[8] She says of society today: "Late twentieth-century machines have made thoroughly ambiguous the difference between natural and artificial, mind and body, self-developing and externally designed, and many other distinctions that used to apply to organisms and machines. Our machines are disturbingly lively, and we ourselves frighteningly inert."[9] Both cases of the cyborg—biological and cultural—highlight the reality that technology can no longer be thought of as simply tools to be applied, but rather is the environment in which we live and breathe and have our being.

The biological cyborg, in which human beings are literally fused with their technology, is a powerful and often violent portrayal of human beings in their relationship with their own technological proclivity, and one that generates an immediate response. The cultural representation of the cyborg seems more benign because it does not shock through forcing a confrontation with that human agency. However, this less common cultural use of the term highlights the extremely complex network of relationships between human beings and the products of human agency, which is sometimes obscured by the more common imagery of the biological cyborg.

The image of the cyborg, both biological and cultural, and the hybridity it represents, is an ambivalent one in this world of shifting boundaries, where technological manipulation of the world relies upon there being some kind of consistent structure or order to affect, and yet in doing so existing notions of some kind of fixed ordering to the natural world are challenged or reject-ed. As Elaine Graham notes, "Yet to speak of an orderliness to nature, of its integrity as a mediation of divine purpose, is not the same as inferring an immutability to nature which forbids the 'unnatural' interventions of tech-nology or cultural diversity. So we must be ware of attributing to 'nature' a fixity and purpose—or even a homogeneity and determinism—which it does not possess. Human relationships to nature are altogether more com-plex, and appeals to what is 'natural' provide little help when, as in the age of advanced biotechnology, this is the very category which is revealed to be malleable and problematic."[10]

Some scholars, such as the sociologist Brenda Brasher, argue that institu-tional religions such as Christianity, with their dependence upon Scripture full of pastoral and agrarian imagery, will struggle to address this world of contemporary technology, much less the cyborg. At one level, religion must respond to the existential questions of the age—to boundary questions such as life and death, gender, bodily augmentation, and transgenic modification that are created in light of new technologies. Additionally, religion must also address the issue of how human beings should live, through the creation of symbols, stories, and images that describe the world and life-giving behavior within it.[11]

This problem is exacerbated, Brasher claims, by the assumptions that underpin traditional interpretations, such as fixed physical embodiment, because for the cyborg,

> universal embodiment is not the defining situation. Instead, embodiment is a preeminent moral question as selves ambiguously colonized by technological tools confront unique border quandaries: concerns about the quantity and quality of their humanity in light of their symbiotic relationship to technology, ambiguity over the loss of self that follows fusion with technology, the challenge of cyborg intimacy, confusion over techno-blurred boundaries of life and death, worry over the vague duplicity involved in spending eight-plus hours a day watching televisions or a computer monitor in contrast to an average of four minutes a day conversing with one's partner or children, sins such as disembodiedness, data lust, flaming, cracking, releasing viruses, excessive upgrading.[12]

Moreover, Brasher argues that sociologically religious communities may just be unwilling to reinterpret their symbols and assumptions in light of emerging categories.[13] So, whereas theological engagement with the cyborg might be possible using restructured anthropologies, the religious commu-nity may not be willing to use such developments. The response may be one of complete withdrawal from engagement, or perhaps a more combative approach that focuses anxiously upon the figure of the cyborg.[14] Certainly the following response to optimistic views about the malleability of human bodies in light of genetic engineering and nanotechnology has a certain stridency: "Can't see the problem? Well, when Jesus returns—Jesus the incarnate Son of God, the first-century Palestinian Jew, his flesh and blood glorified but still his own—when he returns in power and glory to call us to account, what will he find? Will he find faith upon the earth? Will he even find men and women? Or will he say, as he searches for fellow members of *Homo sapiens*, the species he made in his image and took to be his own, and meets self-invented, designer beings, quite literally, 'I never knew you'?"[15]

At its heart, this is Deane-Drummond's "conflicting ontologies of the person" occurring in the "politics of everyday life." It is a clash that is particularly jarring for those within communities who see an inherent static order established in the world that is being challenged by technology. According to Brian Edgar, "Many people find the elimination of these distinctions particularly threatening. Cyborgs—human-machines—are thus seen, perhaps more intuitively than anything, as both dehumanising and a threat to the order of the world. The idea produces existential feelings of insecurity and disorder as though the structure and fabric of society was under threat."[16] Thus the cyborg is seen as part of the same forces that seek to reshape things like traditional understandings of gender, family, and sexuality, and it is also seen as a rejection of conservative views of the immutability of species that forms part of particular "creationist" views of the world. This latter point is a helpful example of Brasher's sociological concern, whereby the assumption of a static creation by a community will not allow the reinterpretation of religious concepts to allow for a more dynamic, or even evolutionary, worldview such as the one Edgar proposes: "We certainly need a theology of species and transformation because whether we view ourselves as a created co-creator or not, new possibilities are facing us. We are certainly approaching a radically new point in history and we possess new powers and the ability to transform humanity."[17] For Brasher, such a theology needs to include the metaphor of the cyborg, because it accurately describes human beings immersed in technology and in doing so it alerts us to the world that humanity inhabits.

Furthermore, the metaphor stands against perspectives that divide the world into overly simplistic dualisms and hierarchies that are used by those in power to maintain control. The cyborg takes within itself these dualisms between inorganic and organic, human and nonhuman, male and female, and holds them in a tension that creates an integral identity. The barriers between the self and the world are lowered, and the connections with the world and those in it are strengthened, as Brasher explains: "Presuming an inseparable connection between the self and other, the cyborg offers a meta-phoric platform upon which complex human identities might be developed whose connective links could stretch out like the World Wide Web itself to embrace and encompass the world. Because it directly faces and accepts the material components of human life, the cyborg as a root metaphor for contemporary human identity offers the capacity to encourage a responsible awareness of and interaction with the material world."[18]

However, to claim that religious traditions, and Christianity in particular, are inflexible systems that do not have the resources to grapple with the figure of the cyborg, as Brasher does, is untrue. The cyborg, by definition, is a figure of hybridity, and the Christian tradition has within it a range of sources that deal with ambiguity and possibility within the notion of the hybrid. These might be drawn upon, together with other strands such as those related to social justice, to provide hope for life within contemporary technoculture.

Hybridity within the Christian Tradition

Examples of hybridity within the Christian tradition include the understand-ing of God as triune; the paradox of the Incarnation that unites Jesus Christ's human and divine natures in hypostatic union; eschatological frameworks that see the Kingdom of God as inaugurated, yet awaiting fullness; tensions between sin and grace in individuals and communities; and anthropologies that see human beings as occupying ambiguous or contested spaces between the categories of matter and spirit, as well as in bearing the *imago Dei*. In what follows, I call attention to the hybridity that is deeply embedded in core Christian beliefs, from the Trinity to the *imago Dei* to the divine/human natures of the incarnate Christ.

Trinity and Hybridity

If an essential feature of the cyborg metaphor is "an inseparable connection between the self and other," then the Christian understanding of God as triune may have something to offer in the way of language to contribute to that exchange. For example, Samuel Powell, reflecting on the character of divine life, sees the call for creatures to participate in the internal life of the triune Godhead as a conversation of difference and identity, forged through the mysterious union of the dissimilar partners of finite and infinite beings, leading to a new sense of identity.[19]

Reflection on these interactions between God, creature, and creation might in turn provide models and analogies useful for grappling with some aspects of the hybrid. One example might be the perichoretic model, seen since the fourth century as describing the mutual interpenetration and indwelling among the threefold identities (or hypostases) within the unbroken unity of the Trinity, and which could be an apt description for elements of cyborg proposals. However, while this perichoretic relationship has sometimes been likened in the past to a dance of pure love, the human relationship with technology might be likened to Susan White's increasingly frantic "dance of delight and dread."[20] An understanding of what a true perichoretic relationship looks like, where each party mutually respects each other out of love, may provide some insight into how to act in the face of technological hybridity and its results. Furthermore, this model of mutual interpenetration and interdependence also has a resonance with the idea of technology as ecology with various networked entities and forces.

Anthropological Hybridity

Themes of hybridity also weave their way through traditional Christian perspectives on human nature, including the tensions between sin and grace in individuals and communities and anthropologies that see human beings as occupying ambiguous or contested spaces between the categories of matter and spirit. The motif of the *imago Dei* is a significant example of anthropological hybridity, in which the finite human creature seems to straddle categories and kinds by virtue of bearing the divine image. On one hand, the human being is firmly integrated into the natural world, whereas on the other, this same finite creature is called to somehow represent the divine to the world. Human beings image a God who creates and re-creates, and human beings play a role transforming creation, and even inject novelty into the world, by exercising their capacities in areas such as art, science, and technology.

This predominantly functional way of understanding the *imago Dei* has been appropriated within contexts that involve engaging with technology through the theological metaphor of human beings as "created co-creators."[21] The "created" aspect of the metaphor asserts the creaturehood of the human being as caused, created, dependent, finite, and not self-generating. The second aspect—"cocreator"—speaks of a calling to act as an agent within the natural world. The finite human being is an agent working with, and for, God, simultaneously mediating the biological, cultural, and also in some way, the spiritual. The metaphor is not without its detractors, particularly those critics who see it as elevating the "cocreation" aspect of the human being above that of the "created" aspect. However, it does serve as a useful example of a theological hybridity through its combination of finitude and freedom, which highlights the two key aspects present in functional interpretations of the *imago Dei* that intersect with technological activity.

Philip Hefner has taken this idea of the human being as created cocreator, a dual-natured crosser of boundaries, and argued that it corresponds closely with the idea of the cyborg. Donna Haraway's definition of cyborgs as "creatures simultaneously animal and machine, who populate worlds ambiguously natural and crafted," and her assertion that "we are all chimeras, theorized and fabricated hybrids of machine and organism; in short, we are cyborgs," inspires Hefner to connect the motifs of cyborg and created cocreator.[22] Just as the cyborg transgresses the boundary between human and technology, and in doing so opens up possibilities of both wonder and anxiety, so the created cocreator fuses the created with itself as creator.[23]

Anne Kull also pursues this correlation between the cyborg and the created cocreator, which occurs when "nature and culture implode in the embodied entities of the world, such as gene, chip, ecosystem, and brain." This leads to the technocultural environment becoming a shifting, dynamic world that raises the questions: Who are our kindred in this world of hybrids, and what kind of livable world are we trying to build?[24] It is within this uncertain world of constant negotiation that cocreation occurs. This cocreation of nature occurs though through the dynamic interaction of humans, nonhumans, and machines, and it thereby allows human creativeness to be affirmed while alerting us to the creativity of the rest of nature.

Christological Hybridity

For Kull, however, it is Jesus Christ who becomes the ultimate cyborg, representing the breaking of boundaries in the fusion of the divine and human, in a manner that defies definition. In this world of hybridity, Christ shows how to balance a constructed nature that fuses distinct worlds, and he calls us to move beyond limited definitions of humanity and divinity.[25] The assertion that God became "enfleshed" in the person of Jesus of Nazareth, the Incarnation, is a paradox of hybrid existence. In Jesus Christ both human and divine natures were united in a hypostatic union that brought together two different realities and held them in tension as a unified identity.

This affirmation, grounded in the Christological orthodoxy of the Creed of Chalcedon, does not seek to explain the actual dynamics between the human and divine nature, but it forms the basic Christological understanding within most of the Christian world. In a hybrid tension, the source of salvation finds its locus in both the divine and human natures present in Jesus. The singular identity of Jesus Christ is found in his functioning always as divinity–humanity, where each of the natures of his being did not function independently of the other and yet are seen to be distinct. In some ways, this is analogous to the concept of the created cocreator, where cocreativity and createdness can be identified distinctly but function as a whole.

The hypostatic union seen in the Incarnation is useful, Kull contends, for engaging with technocultural narratives about what it means to be truly human. As noted above, Kull states that the Incarnation is a nexus that holds various worlds together in a construction. It resists the temptation to reduce everything to either the material or spiritual, and in doing so to assert that a certain vision of humanity is normative. Christ demonstrates the hope that exists when identity is forged out of differences held in dynamic tension, while showing in his death the danger present in those who cannot grasp this tension.

It is in the Incarnation that what is normative becomes visible. God enters into the ordinary, like us and yet unlike us, and "true humanity" is then measured against this. In doing this Christ demonstrates that true embodiment is a matter of choice and freedom that involves, in part, challenging questions about the limits and fates of the body. Thus, for Kull, the concept of the cyborg alerts us to that fact that "we do not have a clearly defined, exhaustive concept of humanity, let alone divinity."[26]

Thus, in a place where ontologies clash, Kull argues that we need to return to consider Jesus Christ—the one who chose to hold mutually exclusive realities in a dynamic tension. His example in life, death, and resurrection then serves as useful in engaging with hybridity for, by "deliberately posing as a hybrid creature, Jesus can show the arbitrariness and constructed nature of what is considered the norm(al)—and often, significantly, natural."[27] For Kull, Jesus Christ as hybrid provides some norm by which humanity, or at least personhood, might be measured. Specifically, the process of being transformed into the *imago Christi* might make it possible to more wholesomely hold in tension the hybridity found in human existence.[28]

In relation to optimistic visions of a technologically supported posthuman existence, such as transhumanism, Kull argues that the figure of Jesus Christ serves to critique two different aspects of those visions. First, she asserts that the Incarnation as cyborg stands against those who would want to flee from the fleshly body and choose an incorporeal existence. Embodiment matters, and those who choose to celebrate the flesh as part of their being should not be denigrated. Second, however, she also rejects the vision of those who see embodiment as all there is, precisely because the Incarnation is at once both hybrid, bodily existence and also transcendence. Together, both elements of transcendence and embodiment are to be celebrated and woven into a whole.[29]

However, directly equating the Incarnation with the cyborg, as Kull does, may not be palatable for those following a strict Chalcedonian understanding of the Incarnation. In this understanding Christ is seen as dual-natured, yet these natures were without confusion, change, division, or separation, and the distinctive properties of each nature are maintained in the one person of

Christ. Thus in Chalcedonian terms, the Incarnation stands as a paradox of distinct yet unified natures, whereas the cyborg's natures are, perhaps, fused indistinguishably into a single, new, hybrid amalgam. As such, within the Christian tradition, competing narratives of the Incarnation may also generate competing narratives of the cyborg.

Eschatological Hybridity

Within an eschatological framework, the hybridity required in the task of standing between two worlds is clearly apparent. The Christian tradition sees the resurrection of Jesus Christ as an act of new creation that will be consummated in fullness at the eschaton. In the meantime, the world exists in an expectant tension, seen particularly in inaugurated eschatologies of the Kingdom of God. Jesus Christ has ushered in the redemptive power of God into creation in a new way, but the fullness of this power will not be revealed or realized until God's purposes for the history of the world are brought to fulfillment and the new Heaven and new Earth meet.

A similar concept that blends Heaven and Earth is that of believers being considered "citizens of Heaven," even though their daily lives are spent upon within the created world (Phil 3:20). In a similar manner to Roman colonists, who were citizens of Rome and yet lived in other parts of the empire, so too the readers of the Letter to the Philippians were to consider themselves inhabitants of one place while also possessing citizenship in another Kingdom. Furthermore, the claim in the Letter to the Galatians that in Christ there is "neither Jew nor Greek, slave nor free, male nor female" (Gal 3:28) is another example of identity being forged out of the internalization of dualisms, in much the same way as the cyborg. The categories of gender, race, and class do not cease to exist in one world, but they do in another—leading to a tension in the borderlands where it is Christ who defines their identity.

Being Hopeful?

These examples of hybridity running through the Christian faith tradition stand against the claims of Brasher and others that Christianity has few or no resources to draw upon in the face of the cyborg. Rather, the Christian tradition has a rich history of engaging with and developing concepts that are hybrid and ambiguous in nature. As such, there are deep traditions—not only of these ideas but also of how Christian communities have wrestled both positively and negatively with issues of hybridity in their history—that provide a foundation for grappling with the cyborg. Of course one might need to find new symbols and languages to do so—as opposed to using the biblical agrarian imagery, for example—but that is not an unusual task in theological reflection and articulation. This is one source of hope, perhaps, for the Christian community.

Second, the narratives of hybridity within the Christian tradition do not stand alone. Rather, they are caught up in a web of relationships with other theological themes and motifs from within the tradition. The functional interpretation of the *imago Dei*, for example, is not just an example of hybridity but also carries within it ethical dimensions stressing human presence as one dimension of God's representation within creation, coupled with a calling to wholesome activity. This agency might then intersect with the prophetic tradition, with its call to social justice and human activity that is concerned with emulating God's concern for the other.

These themes and symbols, when brought into dialogue with the figure of the cyborg and the technoculture that it represents, might give Christians today both the language and motivation to act creatively, transformatively, and redemptively. If indeed it is true that in our everyday lives we are colonized by technology, becoming various forms of cultural and biological cyborgs, then questions about what technology is appropriate come to the fore. One description of how we are bathed in technology and how we might respond is offered by Ian Barbour, who speaks of our search for a "creative technology that is economically productive, ecologically sound, socially just, and personally fulfilling."[30] The themes mentioned above provide some of the theological starting points for following through with this search, for it is precisely though the sort of communitarian dimension that theology provides that we will be able to move the discussion away from a tendency toward individualism.

Where, then, should hope be found in the face of the technological apprehension raised by the image of the cyborg? If to be human is to bear God's image and likeness, then hope is to be found in this calling. The *imago Dei*, seen through the metaphors such as the created cocreator, contains within it explanations of human beings as inherently technological and offers a hint of a trajectory that human technological agency should take. As such, it provides answers to the existential questions that arise out of apprehension's wonder and anxiety, and also provides wisdom for living within technoculture. In particular, it contains an understanding of the interdependent, embodied relationships in which humanity is caught up in the natural world; of a call to agency that does not dehumanize or marginalize others; of the imperative toward beneficent agency, while also recognizing potential for maleficence; and of a recognition that human activity, while questing for the transcendent, is still rooted in the finite.

This understanding, and the others suggested above, provide examples of the richness of language and symbols concerning hybridity found in the

Christian tradition, allowing these answers to be framed using the language of the cyborg and the hybrid present within technocultural discourse.

The presence of narratives of hope does not—and should not—eliminate the narratives of apprehension present within contemporary technoculture. Hope arises from the theological reflection of the tension between wonder and anxiety, as each informs the other, and drives to the fore essential questions about human technological agency. It is essential to have avenues—in communities of faith, in the academy, and in the public square—for raising, discussing, and answering these questions so as to provide hope in the face of this tension between awe and anxiety. Narratives of hope do not displace those of apprehension but rather exist in symbiosis, which allows apprehension to serve a positive purpose in society. Thus the narrative of apprehension generated by public unease about something like genetically modified foods need not lead to futile acceptance of the situation but can instead energize those affected to examine why both wonder and anxiety are raised, and to act in ways that seek to bring about wholeness in that situation. When these things are considered, then there is the possibility of our dwelling hopefully in the borderlands of contemporary technoculture. If human beings, bearers of the *imago Dei*, are indeed "natural-born cyborgs," image bearers situated in hybridity, then the twin narratives of apprehension and hope can aid in securing our hybrid identity, which will lead to human agency that is just, compassionate, and humble before God. In doing so, there is a very real possibility that we can live as "hopeful cyborgs."

Notes

1. Bostrom, "Transhumanist FAQ," §1.1.
2. Robert and Baylis, "Crossing Species Boundaries," 10.
3. Green, *Technoculture*, 167.
4. Deane-Drummond, Grove-White, and Szerszynski, "Genetically Modified Theology," 27. See also Lassen and Jamison, "Genetic Technologies Meet the Public."
5. Clynes and Kline, "Cyborgs and Space."
6. Clark, *Natural-Born Cyborgs*, 3. This way of viewing a human being's interaction with technology is similar to that proposed by Gregory Stock, who argues that human beings are "fyborgs" (functional cyborgs), where technology is fused functionally, rather than physically, with the human person. The latter does occur in some instances, such as dental fillings, pacemakers, and artificial heart valves, but the issue is whether a technology is considered functionally part of the person. See Stock, *Redesigning Humans*, 24–27.
7. Clark, *Natural-Born Cyborgs*, 27–28.
8. Haraway, "Cyborg Manifesto," 291–95.

9. Ibid., 293–94.

10. Graham, "Bioethics after Posthumanism," 184–85.

11. Brasher, *Give Me That Online Religion*, 151–56.

12. Brasher, "Thoughts on the Status of the Cyborg," 817–18.

13. Ibid., 818–19.

14. Hook, "Techno Sapiens Are Coming." Though Hook calls for Christians to engage with technology and to work to see it used to serve the public good, the article's headline plays upon the negative anxieties around the figure of the cyborg.

15. Cameron, "Pursuit of Enhancement."

16. Edgar, "God, Persons and Machines."

17. Ibid.

18. Brasher, "Thoughts on the Status of the Cyborg," 825.

19. Powell, *Participating in God*, 55–57. This type of participation is a calling for all creatures to respond according to their essence. Powell notes that it is a more universal mode of being than soteriological participation in Christ linked more explicitly to redemption, though there is some overlap.

20. White, *Christian Worship*, 18.

21. Hefner, *Human Factor*.

22. Haraway, "Cyborg Manifesto," 291–92.

23. See Hefner, "Created Co-Creator Meets Cyborg, Part One"; and Hefner, "Created Co-Creator Meets Cyborg, Part Two."

24. Kull, "Cyborg Embodiment," 279–80.

25. Ibid., 283.

26. Ibid., 283–84.

27. Ibid., 284.

28. The Eastern concept of *theosis*, and the Protestant one of sanctification, might be seen as processes in this form of hybridity. The human creature can never become God, who is a totally other category, but the divine world can meet the material world in a union that creates a new hybrid creature.

29. Kull, "Cyborg Embodiment," 283.

30. Barbour, *Ethics*, 25.

References

Barbour, Ian G. *Ethics in an Age of Technology: The Gifford Lectures 1989–1991*, vol. 2. San Francisco: HarperSanFrancisco, 1993.

Bostrom, Nick. "The Transhumanist FAQ: A General Introduction." World Transhumanist Association, www.transhumanism.org/resources/FAQv21.pdf.

Brasher, Brenda E. *Give Me That Online Religion*. New Brunswick, NJ: Rutgers University Press, 2004.

———. "Thoughts on the Status of the Cyborg: On Technological Socialization and Its Link to the Religious Function of Popular Culture." *Journal of the American Academy of Religion* 64, no. 4 (1996): 817–18.

Cameron, Nigel M. de S. "The Pursuit of Enhancement: The Latest from Brave New Britain." *Christianity Today*. www.christianitytoday.com/ct/2006/108/32.0.html.

Clark, Andy. *Natural-Born Cyborgs: Minds, Technologies, and the Future of Human Intelligence.* New York: Oxford University Press, 2003.

Clynes, Manfred E., and Nathan S. Kline. "Cyborgs and Space." In *The Cyborg Handbook*, edited by Chris Hables Gray. New York: Routledge, 1995.

Deane-Drummond, Celia, Robin Grove-White, and Bronislaw Szerszynski. "Genetically Modified Theology: The Religious Dimensions of Public Concerns about Agricultural Biotechnology." *Studies in Christian Ethics* 14, no. 2 (2001): 27.

Edgar, Brian. "God, Persons and Machines: Theological Reflections." Institute for the Study of Christianity in an Age of Science and Technology. www.iscast.org.au/pdf/GodPersonsMachines[1].pdf.

Graham, Elaine. "Bioethics after Posthumanism: Natural Law, Communicative Action and the Problem of Self-Design." *Ecotheology* 9, no. 2 (2004): 184–85.

Green, Lelia. *Technoculture: From Alphabet to Cybersex.* Crowsnest, Australia: Allen and Unwin, 2002.

Haraway, Donna. "A Cyborg Manifesto: Science, Technology and Socialist-Feminism in the Late Twentieth Century." In *The Cybercultures Reader*, edited by David Bell and Barbara M. Kennedy. London: Routledge, 2000.

Hefner, Philip. "The Created Co-Creator Meets Cyborg, Part One." Metanexus Institute. www.metanexus.net/metanexus_online/show_article2.asp?ID=8780.

———. "The Created Co-Creator Meets Cyborg, Part Two." Metanexus Institute, www.metanexus.net/metanexus_online/show_article2.asp?ID=8787.

———. *The Human Factor: Evolution, Culture and Religion*, Theology and the Sciences Series. Minneapolis: Fortress Press, 1993.

Hook, C. Christopher. "The Techno Sapiens Are Coming." *Christianity Today* 48, no. 1 (2004).

Kull, Anne. "Cyborg Embodiment and the Incarnation." *Currents in Theology and Mission* 28, nos. 3–4 (2001): 279–80.

Lassen, Jesper, and Andrew Jamison. "Genetic Technologies Meet the Public: The Discourses of Concern." *Science, Technology, & Human Values* 31, no. 1 (2006): 8–28.

Powell, Samuel M. *Participating in God: Creation and Trinity*, Theology and the Sciences Series. Minneapolis: Fortress Press, 2003.

Robert, Jason Scott, and Françoise Baylis. "Crossing Species Boundaries." *American Journal of Bioethics* 3 no. 3 (2003): 1–13.

Stock, Gregory. *Redesigning Humans: Choosing Our Children's Genes.* London: Profile, 2002.

White, Susan. *Christian Worship and Technological Change.* Nashville: Abingdon Press, 1994.

Chapter Seven

Artificial Wombs and Cyborg Births

Postgenderism and Theology

J. JEANINE THWEATT-BATES

What is a "posthuman"? In a sense, it is impossible to define this term, because the posthuman is not one single thing but rather a whole set of possible things.[1] One posthuman possibility is the feminist cyborg, first described by Donna Haraway in her landmark essay referred to in shorthand as the "Cyborg Manifesto." The cyborg, as an organic–mechanical hybrid, functions for Haraway and other "cyberfeminists" as a symbol of the ways in which (post)human bodies often defy our assumptions about what does, and does not, count as natural and as human.[2] Other possibilities are offered by transhumanism, an organized international movement unified in its advocacy of technology to ameliorate, and perhaps transcend, the limitations of the human condition into a state of existence that is "better than well." Nick Bostrom writes that posthumans could be completely synthetic artificial intelligences, enhanced uploaded consciousnesses, or the result of making many smaller but cumulatively profound augmentations to a biological human.[3]

In this chapter I hope to conclusively demonstrate the significant differences between the cyborg and transhumanist posthuman visions, despite the accepted common wisdom whereby the cyborg is categorized as a subset of transhumanist thought. Most important, even when speaking of the "smaller but cumulatively profound augmentations to the biological human," the transhumanists tend to embrace an anthropological dualism, whereas the "cyberfeminists" embrace a strong materialism. To this end, I argue that gender, as an aspect of (post)human embodiment, is one site where these posthuman discourses dramatically diverge. Finally, I suggest that the fact that those engaged in doing Christian theological anthropology have recently begun to appreciate that embodiment opens the door to a theological understanding of the posthuman, one that aligns closely with the feminist cyborg posthuman vision, and that therefore might helpfully critique the problematic aspects of transhumanist anthropology, including gender.

The "Human" in Transhumanism

Despite the admitted diversity of what has become known as the trans-humanist movement, transhumanist activists as different as Nick Bostrom, Simon Young, and James Hughes, along with critics of the movement such as N. Katherine Hayles and Elaine Graham, characterize transhumanism as an extension of Enlightenment humanism.[4] Bostrom writes: "Humanists believe . . . we can make things better by promoting rational thinking, free-dom, tolerance, democracy, and concern for our fellow human beings. . . . Just as we use rational means to improve the human condition and the exter-nal world, we can also use such means to improve ourselves, the human organism . . . technological means that will eventually enable us to move beyond what some would think of as 'human'."[5] As an extension of human-ism, transhumanism broadens the Enlightenment locus of social and his-torical progress to include the biological human organism, and it likewise broadens the rational means whereby this is accomplished to include poten-tial and future technologies.

The category of the human within transhumanist thought remains remarkably continuous with the human of its philosophical antecedent, Enlightenment humanism. The qualities identified as most essentially human in Enlightenment humanism—rationality, autonomy—are proper-ties of the mind, and, conceived as such, disembodied. As Bostrom puts it, "It is not our human shape or the details of our current human biology that define what is valuable about us, but rather our aspirations and ideals, our experiences, and the kinds of lives we lead."[6]

Transhumanist improvements of the biological human organism are gen-erally those that would enable fuller, broader expression of precisely those qualities of mind valorized by Enlightenment humanism; the human body is important only insofar as it enables or hinders the expression of those quint-essential human aspirations, ideals, and experiences. Although transhuman-ists differ in their evaluations of specific improvements, the major goals of transhumanism—extended life or immortality, increased intelligence, true artificial intelligence, uploading consciousnesses—can all be seen as expres-sions of an anthropology that sees the human biological organism as inher-ently flawed and in need of improvement, so that what is valuable about the human may be made more fully manifest. Thus, not only is the human in transhumanism continuous with Enlightenment anthropology, the posthu-man is as well. The transhumanist posthuman is the Enlightenment human, plus: H+.[7]

Gendered Bodies and Postgendered Minds

Gender, as a specific embodied reality, is seen by some transhumanists as "an arbitrary and unnecessary limitation on human potential."[8] George Dvorsky and James Hughes offer a detailed vision of the transcendence of the biologically rooted injustices of gender, through advances in neurotechnology, biotechnology, and reproductive technologies. Of particular importance, Hughes and Dvorsky contend that only a material reengineering of the human biological basis of gender can succeed in truly eliminating the deleterious social effects of patriarchy and heterosexism. The problems of gender inequality and heterosexism reside not primarily in the social but in the biological realm—not in human relationships but in the human body. The solution must therefore be not simply social but also biological. This is the ameliorative role of technology: to reshape the human body in ways that prevent the unjust and oppressive consequences of biological gender. Hughes and Dvorsky write: "Only the blurring and erosion of biological sex, of the gendering of the brain, and of binary social roles by emerging technologies will enable individuals to access all human potentials and experiences regardless of their born sex or assumed gender."[9]

Hughes and Dvorsky's postgender proposal seeks to split the difference between the existing philosophical dichotomy of biological-essentialist and social-constructivist views of gender.[10] By "biological-essentialist," I mean views that women share an innate, fixed, and unchangeable specifically "female nature," grounded in female biology. And by "social constructivist," I mean views, often associated with or based upon the work of Judith Butler, that gender is a socially constructed concept, whereby "woman" is framed in opposition to "man," which then produces an assumption of normative, complementary heterosexual male and female natures.[11] Hughes and Dvorsky argue that *both* social reform and biotechnological transformation are required, as they contend that both female biology and social structures are problematic.

However, by locating the source of the social problem of unequal gender roles in biological "sexual dimorphisms," and by insisting that biological transformation must precede social transformation, Hughes and Dvorsky implicitly grant the biological essentialism they claim to transcend. If it were the case that biological sex did not imply gender essentialism, biological modification would not be necessary. To claim that biological gendering necessarily constrains or limits the potential development of the human person is a kind of inverted essentialism, whereby the biological traits seen as formative for a gendered identity are resented rather than celebrated.

How, then, do Hughes and Dvorsky see themselves as transcending biological essentialism? The key is the basic transhumanist belief in the promise of technology to transcend biological givens—in this case, biological sex
and gender. Gender is a bodily reality that does not ontologically define the
human person, as essentialists would contend; rather, gender is a bodily reality that negatively limits the full potential of the human person. This view
of gender as a bodily reality that constrains or limits but does not define the
person can only make sense within the dualism of transhumanist anthropology, as inherited from its Enlightenment humanist roots. The body, even
when it makes a (negative) difference in the formation of personhood, as
Hughes and Dvorsky argue that gender currently does, is not ontologically
definitive. Technology can, and should, intervene and dispel the illusion of
the ontological necessity and givenness of gender—in effect creating a space
between the human person and the body's gender.

Within this technologically mediated space, the deliberate selection of
desirable, isolated gender traits can then be theoretically envisioned. As
Hughes and Dvorsky write, "Postgenderists do not call for the end of all
gender traits, or universal androgyny, but rather that those traits become a
matter of choice. Bodies and personalities in our postgender future will no
longer be constrained and circumscribed by gendered traits, but enriched by
their use in the palette of diverse self-expression."[12] The goal of postgenderism is enhanced control over the body, by multiplying the possibilities for
self-determined human sexual expression—the ultimate in cross-dressing,
perhaps, whereby biological traits may be assumed and discarded at will, like
items of clothing.[13]

Implicit in this description of the postgender future, however, is the
assumption that gender traits are being freely chosen in a context where
persons have already been freed from the biological imperative of unchosen gender traits. The proliferation of possible gender configurations, then,
is a second moment that depends upon first achieving a biologically non-
gendered, neutral state from which choice can be made, as an expression
of the person's conscious control over the biological body. In fact, Hughes
and Dvorsky acknowledge as much in their abstract, writing that "greater
biological fluidity and psychological androgyny will allow future persons to
explore both masculine and feminine aspects of personality."[14] Despite their
overt rejection of universal androgyny as a postgender goal, then, psychological androgyny functions as a prerequisite to the diverse self-expression
that Hughes and Dvorsky envision. In the transhumanist postgender future,
bodies may indeed be multiply gendered, but persons will not be.

Further, the potential proliferation of multiple genders arises from idiosyncratic and individually determined combinations of traits that are still

categorically binary, either "masculine" or "feminine." At this point, the biological problem has theoretically been technologically solved, but the social constructs exist unchanged. Worse, however, despite the authors' apparent intent, is the way in which these binary gender categories still function to signal masculine traits as positive, and feminine traits as negative.

This is seen with particular clarity in Hughes's discussion of artificial wombs. Though "patriarchal culture contributes," Hughes and Dvorsky argue that gender inequalities are "also the inevitable result of the greater burden of childbearing on women, and the different abilities and aspirations of the gendered brain."[15] Eventually, therefore, artificial wombs "will be attractive for all women, as an alternative to the burdens and risks of pregnancy and delivery, and to allow a level of control, purity and optimization of the uterine environment impossible in a woman's body."[16] The possibility that biological wombs might be superior to a technological alternative, or that pregnancy and birth might be experienced by women as desirable rather than burdensome and risky, is apparently unthinkable. Rather than proposing a solution to these social inequalities in the form of social policies that honor these aspects of female embodiment, the solution is to reengineer these problematic female bodies. The benefit of artificial wombs is the elimination of the problematic embodied reality of pregnancy and childbirth, which thereby allows women's bodies to function more like men's bodies—an *andro*gynous postgender future indeed.

Cyborg Gender and Postgender

In both the coauthored "postgenderism" paper and in Hughes's monograph *Citizen Cyborg*, Donna Haraway's now-famous "Cyborg Manifesto" is cited as evidence of "a transhumanist ideological thread that has grown in academia."[17] Hughes interprets Haraway's presentation of the cyborg as "a new liberatory androgynous archetype, [in which] we can find liberation from patriarchy and capitalism."[18] However, Hughes misses crucial aspects of Haraway's feminist cyborg project that oppose this vision of transhumanist postgenderism: her emphasis on embodiment, her ambivalence toward technology, and, most important for this discussion, her rejection of androgyny as an ideal.

In the "Cyborg Manifesto," Haraway says "no" to both Enlightenment anthropology and its mirror twin, reactionary feminist gender essentialism. On both sides, the identity of woman qua woman is assumed to be natural, self-evident, and unchanging—whether this is seen as a deficiency or as something to be celebrated. Saying "no" to Enlightenment anthropology—which defines the human in terms of rationality and autonomy—is not necessarily to say "yes" to the category of Woman, which itself is a product of Enlightenment anthropology, the ontological counterpart of Man. Identifying herself as "cyborg" becomes Haraway's symbolic shorthand for the rejection of any attempt to define human identity on the basis of "nature." This basic stance is the key to Haraway's posthuman discourse, whereby she breaks down the dichotomy between nature and culture, or nature and technology.

Because the cyborg is neither wholly organic nor solely mechanical, it straddles these taken-for-granted ontological and social categories. It is this hybridly embodied aspect of the cyborg's existence that simultaneously holds so much threat and promise. Human beings construct social categories as a way of ordering our coexistence, and we often experience the transgression of the boundaries of these categories as primordial chaos unleashing itself into our lives. The hybridity of the cyborg is therefore often interpreted as an invasion of the human by the machine, resulting in a loss of free will and autonomy to mechanistic determinism and external control—what Stephen Garner terms "narratives of apprehension."[19] Yet those who find themselves outside the clean definitions of those social categories often experience the transgression of the boundaries as liberation. From this point of view, having never belonged to the Enlightenment "human" category, the cyborg's existence is not simply descriptive of reality but also liberative, as it deconstructs a false and narrow category that has historically functioned to exclude more humans than it has included. The cyborg, then, is also a protagonist in posthuman "narratives of hope."[20]

For Haraway, then, specific, hybrid embodiment is the counter to both the Enlightenment dualism that defines the human as disembodied rationality and also to the biological essentialism of some feminists, as exemplified by discourses on natural childbirth and goddess-talk, that pits the (female) natural against the (male) technological. Haraway never loses sight, therefore, of the importance of embodiment in her development of the cyborg as metaphor.[21] Indeed, without a continuing emphasis on the importance of embodied experience, the cyborg loses its salience as an image. This is a materialism that takes seriously not simply the fact of human embodiment generally but also the specificity of the differences between human bodies and the impact of these differences in defining what it means to be (post) human.

Hughes's techno-optimism contrasts sharply with Haraway's delicate balancing between the oppressive and liberating potentials of the cyborg, an aspect of the "Cyborg Manifesto" that is clearly evident in Haraway's description of the cyborg as "the awful apocalyptic *telos* of the 'West's' escalating dominations of abstract individuation, an ultimate self untied at last from all dependency, a man in space."[22] It is this that makes her appropriation of the cyborg an ironic move; she never forgets this dubious original conception of the cyborg as the ultimate Man, even while she argues that the cyborg, as the "illegitimate offspring" of the Enlightenment, may very well be unfaithful to its origins. Haraway's attitude is a much more guarded and conditional hope, dependent upon the ties of kinship that are recognized and fostered, or not.[23]

Most important, Hughes misinterprets Haraway in claiming the androgyny of the cyborg; Haraway's cyborg is consistently female, "a girl who's trying not to become Woman."[24] Moreover, it is also clear that women are cyborgs (though not necessarily the only cyborgs) precisely as women— creatures who cross over from the wrong side of the ontological tracks, and thus refuse to stay neatly put in their appointed category of other-than-male. This boundary crossing does not make women androgynous, as if somehow the surrender of a particular gender is required in the act of crossing; indeed, from Haraway's point of view, this would be nothing less than the requirement to annihilate identity in the name of a false liberation, a secular version of the Gospel of Thomas's promise to Mary Magdalene that in Heaven she will be saved by being made a man.

The source of this misreading is Hughes's view of gender and postgender through the focal point of the transhumanist inheritance of the Enlightenment view of the body as the property of the individual self. Viewed through this lens, which presupposes a distance between self and body, the androgyny of the mind (the person) can be expressed willfully through deliberate manipulations of the body in idiosyncratic combinations of isolated gender traits. Transhumanist postgenderism is thus another expression of transhumanism's continuity with, in N. Katherine Hayles's phrase, the "liberal humanist subject," resulting in a split of the person from his body. It is exactly this move that Haraway resolutely refuses to make, instead maintaining a consistent materialism that takes seriously the feminist slogan "Our Bodies, Ourselves," even while redefining it through her invocation of the cyborg.[25]

Postgender, therefore, in the transhumanist sense of somehow getting beyond gender entirely, is not a concept that Haraway advocates.[26] In a 2006 interview Haraway comments: "In some ways postgender is a meaningful notion, but I get really nervous about the ways in which it gets made into a utopian project."[27] For her, postgender cannot mean transcendence, denial, or the reconstruction of the material reality of gender. Rather, it means finally getting the fact that our socially constructed gender categories have never fit the material reality of our bodies in the first place. The cyborg is therefore "postgender" in only a limited and very specific sense, in a context where the word "gender" signifies the social construct of essentialized Woman.

On this point, it is instructive to contrast Haraway and Hughes on a specific aspect of female embodiment, that is, wombs and birthing. In the "Cyborg Manifesto," Haraway associates the metaphor of birth and rebirth with the universalizing and essentializing of the maternal Woman. She states, therefore, that cyborgs are about "monstrous regeneration" rather than birth.[28] This has on occasion been interpreted as the exclusion of the maternal from Haraway's cyborg altogether.[29] This would seem to approximate what Hughes advocates in his endorsement of artificial wombs: a liberation from gender that necessitates the rejection of this aspect of female embodiment.

Haraway, however, rejects birth only in the context of biological essentialism; the material reality of birthing is not the problem, but the construction of a universal identity based on it, whereby all women inherit "skill in mothering and its metaphoric extensions."[30] Rejecting the universality of the maternal does not mean rejecting the reality of the maternal; rather, it means recognizing the materiality of birth as cyborg, not universal or natural. Indeed, within a medical context that regularly confuses the natural and technological, birthing is itself (literally) a cyborg process.[31] A womb need not be artificial for birthing to be cyborg! Moreover, the liberation that Hughes sees for women in the artificial womb is the illusory promise of Enlightenment autonomy—a denial of the material, embodied cyborg kinships made so obvious in the process of birth, and that Haraway celebrates as the ironic potential of the cyborg.

In an important sense, then, transhumanist and cyborg views of gender are starkly opposed. Hughes and Dvorsky see binary gender as a problematic, biological, and material reality, which therefore requires a biotechnological solution. Haraway, in contrast, argues passionately that biological, material reality of gendered bodies actually belies the problematic socially constructed binary gender categories. One might sum up this difference by saying that, for Hughes and Dvorsky, our bodies are the problem; but for Haraway, finally paying attention to our bodies is the solution.

Theology and (Post)gender

What, finally, is a theologian to make of this confusing and contradictory discourse on the posthuman, transhumanism, cyborgs, gender, and postgenderism? What does the Christian tradition of theological anthropology have to offer this conversation, and what may we in turn learn from it? What sorts of interdisciplinary theological constructions result from a convergence of Christian theological anthropology and transhumanist postgenderism? What sorts of theological constructions might result from a conversation with the feminist cyborg?

Many critics of transhumanism have claimed that it functions as a covertly religious worldview; a chief exhibit among the supporting evidence for this claim is the disembodied transhumanist anthropology. It is hard to miss the parallel between Neoplatonic Christian theological views of the body as "evil, seductive matter" and the transhumanist view of human biological bodies as placing negative limits on human potential, particularly when articulations of notions of immortality are explicit in both discourses. Even when, as in Hughes and Dvorsky's postgenderism proposal, the goal is to refashion rather than abandon the body, anthropological dualism is a necessary component of the transhumanist vision.

In its conversation with transhumanism, then, the Christian tradition's own historical ambivalence toward the human body becomes an important focal point. In this regard, Elizabeth Moltmann-Wendel asks, "Is the human body a good creation of God? Or evil, seductive matter which one does better to forget, despise, punish, if need be burn, so that the soul or the apparently immortal part of the person is saved?" concluding "that is the problem for Christianity."[32] The recognition of this ambivalence toward the body as a problem explains both the need and motivation for doing "body theology" as a corrective for the dualistic tendency in Christian anthropology.[33] The Christian tradition itself, then, becomes subject to revision in the light of this emphasis on embodiment, and it offers rich sites for theological discussion—for example, the central Christian doctrine of the Incarnation, and the importance of the body in Pauline ecclesiology.

This general retrieval of the importance of embodiment is echoed and intensified by the work of feminist theologians whose critique of the Christian tradition is not simply that the body per se has been ignored but also that the normative human body has historically been identifiably male.[34] Even further, queer theology insists that the material realities of human bodies often defy the social categories of binary gender, and precisely in so doing, function as sites of theological revelation.

The interdisciplinary conversation between Christian theology and transhumanism on the subject of gender, therefore, offers multiple possibilities, of both convergence and critique. If, as in certain classical dualistic strands of Christian anthropology, embodiment is seen as incidental and negative, then a Christian postgenderism might result if one took the view that persons (or, in classical theological language, souls) are not essentially gendered but are only human bodies. This theological anthropology resembles Hughes and

Dvorsky's postgenderism in its assumption of an essential androgyny separate from embodied gender. The anthropological similarity persists, even if the technological means of achieving postgenderism in the here and now were to be rejected on other grounds, as attempts to "play God."

A Christian rejection of postgenderism, conversely, might take the form of arguing that persons (souls) are essentially gendered, drawing upon the discourses of natural kinds and creation. Here it is not an appreciation of embodiment that fuels the rejection of postgenderism but the conviction that men and women are ontologically distinct, and that they have been created thus by God to fill socially distinct, complementary roles—a conviction often at play in the opposition to homosexuality and to opening the ordained ministry to women within certain Christian traditions. From this point of view, pursuing the transhumanist goal of postgenderism would be actively sinful, a rejection of God's creation of binary biological genders.

The fact that those engaged in doing Christian theological anthropology have relatively recently begun to appreciate embodiment, however, prompts a rejection of both transhumanist postgenderism and gender essentialism, precisely because the body itself matters. Paying attention to specific embodiments impels the recognition that "we have constructed bodies within boundaries that could never contain them but have at times distorted and mutilated them."[35] Theological constructions of the human that ignore, or universalize, the body, gender, and sexuality miss the ways in which multiple human embodiments make a difference in our conceptions of the human.

This has been most forcefully articulated within queer theology: "More than anything else," Marcella Althaus-Reid and Lisa Isherwood write, "queer theology is an incarnated, body theology," and this means not simply celebrating a generic embodiment but also a "plunge into flesh in its unrefined fullness in order to embrace and be embraced by the divine."[36] The theological emphasis on the specificity and materiality of the doctrines of the Creation and the Incarnation reiterates, from within the Christian tradition itself, Haraway's basic cyborg insight. Our created, incarnated, bodily selves belie the socially constructed categories of Man, Woman, and the generic universal Human. In this sense, then, queer theology is posthuman theology, or more specifically, cyborg theology—and therefore it is emphatically not a transhumanist postgender theology.

I have argued, perhaps idiosyncratically—but nonetheless, I believe, accurately—that transhumanist postgenderism and the cyborg feminism are different, indeed opposing, posthuman constructions. Yet in many instances Haraway's work is either ignored or characterized as a subset of transhumanist discourse. This poses two problems. First, it implies a misinterpretation of Haraway's cyborg. And second, it misattributes cyborg attitudes to transhumanism. The consequences of such a theological misreading of the posthuman is that Christian theology's contribution to posthuman discourse, and its possible intervention in the construction of the posthuman, is fatally weakened. We may be, as N. Katherine Hayles contends, at an important historical juncture with regard to our emerging posthuman future, and if so, we bear a moral responsibility in envisioning and constructing our future selves. If, indeed, to use Stephen Garner's term, the cyborg is the "hopeful posthuman," then it is crucial to press transhumanists to in*corporate*—pun intended—the insights that Haraway's cyborg has to offer.[37]

Notes

1. For a full argument regarding the inevitable plurality of the posthuman, see Thweatt-Bates, "Cyborg Christ."

2. Haraway, "Cyborg Manifesto."

3. Bostrom, "Transhumanist FAQ." Bostrom notes that "the latter alternative would probably require either the redesign of the human organism using advanced nanotechnology or its radical enhancement using some combination of technologies such as genetic engineering, psychopharmacology, anti-aging therapies, neural interfaces, advanced information management tools, memory enhancing drugs, wearable computers, and cognitive techniques" (pp. 4–5).

4. Ibid.; Graham, *Representation of the Post/Human*; Hayles, *How We Became Posthuman*; Hughes, *Citizen Cyborg*; Hughes, "Transhumanist Politics"; Young, *Designer Evolution*.

5. Bostrom, "Transhumanist FAQ."

6. Ibid.

7. Transhumanism is often abbreviated as "H+." The World Transhumanist Association's recent rebranding as "Humanity Plus" is also a signal, as I see it, of the awareness within the transhumanist movement of the rhetorical need to present the posthuman as continuous, rather than discontinuous, with current notions of the human.

8. Hughes and Dvorsky, "Postgenderism."

9. Ibid., 7.

10. Ibid., 5.

11. See Gardner, "Biological Determinism," "Essentialism," and "Butler, Judith."

12. Hughes and Dvorsky, "Postgenderism," 2.

13. Not coincidentally, N. Katherine Hayles describes this scenario rather differently: "My nightmare is a culture inhabited by posthumans who regard their bodies as fashion accessories"; Hayles, *How We Became Posthuman*, 5.

14. Hughes and Dvorsky, "Postgenderism," 2.

15. Ibid., 3.

16. Hughes, *Citizen Cyborg*, 87.

17. Ibid., 207. Cf. Hughes and Dvorsky, "Postgenderism," 5–6.

18. Hughes and Dvorsky, "Postgenderism." In *Citizen Cyborg*, Hughes adds, "[Haraway] proposes the cyborg as the liberatory mythos for all women"; Hughes,

Citizen Cyborg, 207. In Hughes's defense, he does not appear to be the only one who misses Haraway's point on the material reality of gendered bodies; Mitchell, "Bodies That Matter."

19. Garner, "Transhumanism." For more on Garner's theological assessment of cyborgs, see chapter 6 in this book.

20. Ibid., 257.

21. "These ontologically confusing *bodies*, and the practices that produce specific embodiment, are what we have to address, not the false problem of *dis*embodiment." Haraway, "Fetus," 186.

22. Haraway, "Cyborg Manifesto," 151.

23. Further, the tendency for the cyborg to remain the hypermasculine, militaristic technoborg is evidenced in the host of misinterpretations of Haraway's attempt to use the cyborg as an ironic and subversive figure and the subsequent loss of the feminist and political dimension; see Bastian, "Haraway's Lost Cyborg."

24. Haraway, "Cyborgs at Large," 20.

25. Haraway, "Cyborg Manifesto," 181.

26. In fact, Haraway has explicitly distanced herself from the term "postgender," and also the term "posthuman," feeling that both terms now function to signal concepts that she rejects.

27. Gane and Haraway, "When We Have Never Been Human," 137–38.

28. Haraway, "Cyborg Manifesto," 180.

29. As, e.g., Katharyn Privett's reading: "In an effort to resist maternal essentialism, Haraway creates a material corporeality that excludes the maternal as one possible element in a feminist constituency." Privett, "Sacred Cyborgs," 176–77.

30. Haraway, "Cyborg Manifesto," 180.

31. Mercedes and Thweatt-Bates, "Bound in the Spiral Dance."

32. Moltmann-Wendel, *I Am My Body*, 36.

33. Isherwood and Stuart, *Introducing Body Theology*; Moltmann-Wendel, *I Am My Body*; Nelson, *Body Theology*.

34. See Tobler, "Beyond a Patriarchal God"; and Ruether, *Sexism and God-Talk*.

35. Althaus-Reid and Isherwood, "Thinking Theology," 310.

36. Ibid., 309.

37. Garner, "Transhumanism," 257.

References

Althaus-Reid, Marcella, and Lisa Isherwood. "Thinking Theology and Queer Theory." *Feminist Theology* 15, no. 3 (2007): 302–14.

Bastian, Michelle. "Haraway's Lost Cyborg and the Possibilities of Transversalism." *Signs: Journal of Women in Culture & Society* 31, no. 4 (2006): 1027–49.

Bostrom, Nick. "The Transhumanist FAQ: A General Introduction," 2003. http://transhumanism.org/index.php/WTA/faq/.

Gane, N., and D. Haraway. "When We Have Never Been Human, What Is to Be Done? Interview with Donna Haraway." *Theory Culture & Society* 23, nos. 7–8 (2006): 135–58.

Gardner, Catherine Villanueva. "Biological Determinism," "Essentialism," and "Butler, Judith." In *Historical Dictionary of Feminist Philosophy*. Lanham, MD: Scarecrow Press, 2006.

Garner, Stephen. "Transhumanism and the *Imago Dei*: Narratives of Apprehension and Hope." PhD dissertation, University of Auckland, 2006.

Graham, Elaine. *Representation of the Post/Human: Monsters, Aliens and Others in Popular Culture*. New Brunswick, NJ: Rutgers University Press, 2002.

Haraway, Donna J. "A Cyborg Manifesto: Science, Technology and Socialist-Feminism in the Late Twentieth Century." In *Simians, Cyborgs and Women: The Reinvention of Nature*, 149–81. New York: Routledge, 1991.

———. "Cyborgs at Large: Interview with Donna Haraway." In *Technoculture*, edited by A. Penley and C. Ross, 1–20. Minneapolis: University of Minnesota Press, 1991.

———. "Fetus: The Virtual Speculum in the New World Order." In *Modest_Witness@Second_Millennium.Femaleman©_Meets_Oncomouse™: Feminism and Technoscience*, 173–212. New York: Routledge, 1997.

Hayles, N. K. *How We Became Posthuman: Virtual Bodies in Cybernetics, Literature, and Informatics*. Chicago: University of Chicago Press, 1999.

Hughes, James. *Citizen Cyborg: Why Democratic Societies Must Respond to the Redesigned Human of the Future*. Cambridge, MA: Westview Press, 2004.

———. "Transhumanist Politics, 1700 to the Near Future." *Re-public*. www.re-public.gr/en/?p=638.

Hughes, James, and George Dvorsky. *Postgenderism: Beyond the Gender Binary*. Hartford: Institute for Ethics and Emerging Technologies, 2008.

Isherwood, Lisa, and Elizabeth Stuart. *Introducing Body Theology*. Vol. 2 of *Introductions to Feminist Theology*, edited by Mary Gray, Lisa Isherwood, Catherine Norris, and Janet Wootten. Sheffield: Sheffield Academic Press, 1998.

Mercedes, Anna, and Jennifer Thweatt-Bates. "Bound in the Spiral Dance: Spirituality and Technology in the Third Wave." In *Feminist Spirituality: The Next Generation*, edited by Chris Klassen. Lanham, MD: Lexington Books, 2009.

Mitchell, Kaye. "Bodies That Matter: Science Fiction, Technoculture, and the Gendered Body." *Science Fiction Studies* 33, no. 1 (2006): 109–28.

Moltmann-Wendel, Elizabeth. *I Am My Body: New Ways of Embodiment*, translated by John Bowden. London: SCM Press, 1994.

Nelson, James. *Body Theology*. Louisville: Westminster / John Knox Press, 1992.

Privett, Katharyn. "Sacred Cyborgs and 21st Century Goddesses." *Reconstruction: Studies in Contemporary Culture*, vol. 7, no. 4 (2007). An online journal accessed on July 29, 2011, at http://reconstruction.eserver.org/c74/privett.shtml

Ruether, Rosemary Radford. *Sexism and God-Talk: Toward a Feminist Theology*. Boston: Beacon Press, 1983.

Thweatt-Bates, J. Jeanine. "The Cyborg Christ: Theological Anthropology, Christology, and the Posthuman." PhD dissertation, Princeton Theological Seminary, 2009.

Tobler, Judy. "Beyond a Patriarchal God: Bringing the Transcendent Back to the Body." *Journal of Theology for Southern Africa* 106 (2000): 35–50.

Young, Simon. *Designer Evolution: A Transhumanist Manifesto*. Amherst, NY: Prometheus Books, 2006.

Chapter Eight

Taking Leave of the Animal?

The Theological and Ethical Implications of Transhuman Projects

CELIA DEANE-DRUMMOND

In this chapter I focus on the relationship between transhumanism and what might be termed human "animality" or "creatureliness." I believe that this is important, because taken in isolation the kind of enhancements portrayed by transhuman philosophers might seem relatively innocuous. By drawing particularly on the work of Nick Bostrom, the philosopher and protagonist of transhumanism, I hope to uncover subtle tendencies toward perceiving human development in disembodied terms. This is important for theological anthropology. I argue against any linear historical trajectory from Augustine, through to René Descartes, and from modernity and transhumanism.[1] However, I suggest that patterns of relationships in the thought of Augustine, especially stripped of their theological rootedness in an affirmation of creation, expose a detachment from understanding human beings as grounded in solidarity with other animals through common creaturely being. I suggest that this is important ethically in assessing the trajectory of transhumanism, inasmuch as it shapes how we perceive human flourishing that in turn has an impact on how we treat other human beings and other animals.

Transhuman Enhancements as Transanimal?

The rhetoric associated with transhuman philosophy focuses most commonly on the natural limitations of the human condition and how these might be overcome by various bioengineering technologies. If these are couched in case studies that are illustrative of human suffering and disease, the reader is naturally and readily drawn to sympathize with the use of such technologies. A similar approach may be used in arguments for embryonic stem cell research, for example. The philosopher John Harris argues this case in *Enhancing Evolution*. At the start of the book he puts the case baldly: "Wouldn't it be wonderful if we humans could live longer healthier lives with immunity to many of the diseases like cancer and HIV/AIDS that currently beset us? Even more wonderful might be the possibility of increased mental powers, powers of memory, reasoning and concentration, or the possibility of increased physical powers, strength, stamina, endurance, speed of reaction and the like. Wouldn't it be wonderful?"[2]

Further, when placed in such a context, the difference between therapy and enhancement evoke a blurred line that is hard to maintain, and that therefore is not necessarily useful in ethical analysis. Any resistance to transhumanism when it is couched in terms of resistance to disease or a healthier life, or increased mental or physical powers, might seem reminiscent of Luddite sensibility. Yet perhaps it is important to reflect a little more carefully on the practical implications of what is being suggested. It might seem wonderful in terms of causing us to be amazed, but would it necessarily always be something that humanity always strives after as a good? Harris believes that hostility toward enhancement is misplaced, comparing such changes with socially accepted enhancements such as wearing glasses and immunization. For him the only ethical quandary here is a balance between risk and benefits—do the benefits outweigh any possible risks that might be present; and if these can be managed, then we should go ahead. He also presses for individual freedom of choice and autonomy as another reason why governments need to back such a shift.

Yet Harris goes further than this and presses for such changes as a matter of *obligation* to create a new human future. In this he perceives enhancements fitting in to a view of what might be broadly termed human "evolution," understood as a human construction. He goes as far as to suggest that we need to replace natural selection with deliberate selection and Darwinian evolution with enhancement evolution.[3] He believes, therefore, that the potential of humanity can only be reached by taking such deliberate steps, achieved through enhancement technologies. He also reinforces this by suggesting that there was never a time when humans did not try and improve their lot, as "ape-descended" persons.[4] Here he seems to be using a naturalistic Darwinian argument, that because even our early ancestors were presumably selected to try and improve their situation, then we should do the same. The difference is that now, according to him, evolution is within our powers to manipulate.[5] I suggest that beginning with such an analysis helps to explain the significance of those particular cases of enhancement that seem at first sight to be reasonable and realistic.

Bostrom is an atheist philosopher and transhuman activist who, paradoxically perhaps, has written on the philosophical aspects of global risk taking, as well as promoting his own version of transhuman philosophy.[6] In a manner reminiscent of forecasts made by economists or policymakers, he envisages four scenarios for humanity's future evolution: extinction, recurrent collapse, plateau, and posthumanity. He believes that his own approach builds on what is possible at the moment, rather than being invented through science fiction or theology—which he understands as, for example, just one screen for our hopes and fears, or a means whereby ideology is mobilized.[7] For him, technology drives economic growth; hence, our projections of technology are strongly correlated with human development. His optimistic view of technology leads to a more or less linear development, where all possible human capabilities that can be attained through technology will be attained. He names such a position in grandiose terms as the "Technological Completion Conjecture."[8] Although he refrains from using the word "progress," his observation that each new generation is more "advanced" than its predecessor implies a positive outcome.

He also believes that positive outcomes will happen in one scenario, which he names as the posthuman one. His argument for posthumanism sounds attractive when placed alongside the three other scenarios. The possibility of a plateau, which maintains the status quo, is implausible for him because he believes it is unrealistic.[9] The most important technological developments for him, and for the topic of this chapter, are those that impinge directly on human biology. Here he speaks positively in terms of the control of human senescence, so that life expectancy is about 1,000 years; and happiness is enhanced by the "control of brain circuitry responsible for subjective well being," the use of drugs, and other neurotechnologies in order to adjust "personality, emotional character, mental energy, romantic attachments and moral character. Cognitive enhancements might deepen our intellectual lives."[10] Such developments are, he suggests, within the bounds of physical possibility.[11] There are, however, complexity barriers worth considering, which means that highly complex systems go wrong in unexpected ways, though he is reluctant to admit that this would apply to *all* technologies enabling a posthuman condition. Given, however, the complexity of biological systems, and the areas of ignorance, I remain rather much more skeptical of the possibility that anything like what he terms the "posthuman" condition is achievable. But his definition of what might count as a posthuman condition is characterized by one or more of the following:[12]

1. population greater than 1 trillion,
2. life expectancy greater than 500 years,
3. large fraction of the population with cognitive capacity more than 2 standard deviations above the current human maximum,
4. more or less complete control over sensory inputs for the majority of people most of the time,

5. human psychological suffering is rare, and
6. any change comparable to the above.

Presumably by point 6, he means some other shift in the human condition that might have a similarly drastic impact. An abrupt transition to this state is called the singularity hypothesis, often associated in earlier writing with artificial intelligence.

Whether such changes happen rapidly or gradually is not all that relevant to the present discussion. What matters here are the kinds of scenarios envisaged by those who detach human beings from their sense of being finite creatures rooted in animal desires, fears, and needs. For the purposes of the present discussion, I use the term "transhumanism" to refer to those specific projects that deliberately aim at the kind of scenario envisaged here. There may be more "modest" variants of transhumanism that keep strictly within a limited boundary of enhancement in, for example, resistance to disease. Comparing these kinds of examples with, for example, "natural" ways of promoting disease resistance through diet or exercise is, to my mind at least, underhanded, for it implies that concerns or worries about such technologies are unreasonable.

As we might expect, some of the projected bioengineering technological developments will be tested out on other animals first. This is already happening with the inherited genetic engineering of other animals. Scientists conducting experimental trials with mice have already shown how genetic manipulation can change the ability of mice to memorize and feel fear.[13] Because memory is conserved in evolutionary terms, it is likely that genetically engineered humans would respond in similar ways. Bostrom and his colleague Anders Sandberg did not consider whether such work was justified in live animal subjects, though they did raise the question briefly as to whether other primates might be given enhancements as well, so that they would have a mental intelligence closer to that of humans. This would amount to an argument for a transanimal condition in the sense that now other animals have capacities beyond their normal functioning. What might count in order to make this fully "postanimal" for other animal subjects, in an analogous way to "posthuman," is only a matter of speculation.

The basic idea that humans might be able to enhance other animal species has been around in popular culture for some time. H. G. Wells's classic account in *The Island of Dr Moreau* (1896), or, more chilling perhaps, Pierre Boulle's *La Planète de Singes* (1963) portray fictional accounts of such a scenario. But the serious discussion on the possibility of "uplift" in animals by David Brin's *The Uplift Saga* demonstrates its continuing popularity.[14] The ethical implication of the term "uplift" is positive, but objections to such tampering include whether any such cognitive manipulations will improve the lot of the creatures concerned. Furthermore, the differences in neurology between humans and other primates and its complexity are such that other neurological faculties could not be changed simultaneously, which could lead to morally objectionable scenarios where one capacity might be enhanced but the creature would lack the mental sophistication to deal with such enhancement. Yet I suggest that given the legal strictures on experimentation on human subjects in most jurisdictions, it seems highly likely that the experimental basis for transhumanism will be tested out first through the use of experimental animal subjects. There are also biotechnological developments in animals that are already in place, and these developments pave the way for what might happen in human beings.

Serious discussions of animal biotechnology have received comparatively little philosophical, ethical, and theological attention compared with human biotechnology.[15] One of the reasons for this may be the anthropological bias built into ethical and theological discourse. Another reason may be the concentration of ethical discourse in terms of animal rights, with all forms of biotechnology viewed as an infringement of these rights.[16] Legal regulations may be put in place just to reassure the public and thus be permissive of such science—and this accusation is also true of transhumanism.[17] The idea of inevitability in animal biotechnology, for example, is also latent in transhuman arguments.[18] The difference is that the Kantian imperative to treat people as ends rather than as means to particular ends does not figure in the imagination of most scientists working with other animals, whereas this imperative is enshrined in medical practice in most Western nations. The possibility of abuse of humans or animals no longer able to show memory or fear exists alongside the bald possibility of memory enhancement.

Although advocates of transhumanism recognize what might be termed the "existential risk" of new technologies, analysis that takes the form of a cost/benefit ratio is wedded to a form of consequentialist ethics that assumes legal restraint will be sufficient. Paul Thomson has exposed the weakness of cost/benefit analysis in taking account of the *social* consequences of new animal biotechnologies, and much the same critique can be applied to transhumanism. Part of the problem here is the issue of inevitability, so that "the pattern has been to see technological change as inevitable and to see the problem as one of distributing its benefits and costs; this image treats technological change as if it were an act of God, like a hurricane or an earthquake, and not as something for which human beings or human organizations could be held responsible."[19] Finding out what that task might be in theological terms for an ethics of biotechnology that involves other animals, who share a common theological status as creatures, has yet to be worked out.[20]

The word "postanimal" as applied to animals other than humans may also be understood in a further sense as referring to the trajectory of posthumanity in the manner understood by Bostrom and his collaborators. This is different from what might be termed "cultural" posthumanity that serves to unsettle traditional interpretations of what it means to be human, because the kind of posthumanity that Bostrom advocates is associated with modernity—through science and technology—and seeks to be grounded in that, even while projecting this into future scenarios that seem, to most readers at least, to be speculative rather than residing in concrete technologies.

Are There Theological Antecedents of the Postanimal?

The increasing drive toward technological means to enhance human performance—reinforced by the particular philosophical approach of Bostrom, Harris, and others—raises important theological questions about eschatology—our hopes for the future, as well as how we understand what might be loosely termed "theological anthropology." Though in the past anthropology was seen in its futuristic light through theology, the advent of transhumanism has shifted the agenda, so that now secular discourse includes future projections alongside its discussion of what might count as human flourishing. Yet the kind of human life envisaged by such scenarios is one where the suffering, complexity, and anxiety associated with the contingencies of modern life have largely, if not entirely, faded from view. It offers, then, a form of perfection that is very different from the kind of perfect life recommended by the early church, where the virtues were the goal and measure of human existence.[21]

However, alongside this anthropological strand that stressed the importance of virtues in the Christian life, there was another strand as mediated through the work of Augustine of Hippo. The influence of Plato on Augustine is well known, but what is relevant here is how he interpreted Plato's ideas in his understanding of the specific place and role of humanity. His emphasis, in particular, is on the importance of reason in human beings, such that it distances humanity from other animals. He came back to this issue again and again, refining his ideas over years of reflection on the topic. In one section of his book *On the Literal Interpretation of Genesis*, which remained unfinished, he pressed the case that not everything about humanity was made according to the likeness of God, but only the "rational substance."[22] In a later section he filled this out further, citing Genesis 1.28: "Thus 'Let us make man to our image and likeness' is correctly understood according to what is within man and is his principal part, that is, according to the mind. For the whole of man should be assessed from that which holds the principle place in man and which distinguishes him from the beasts."[23]

Although Augustine recognized that corporate nature has its place—in common with "the cattle," a generic term that he used to mean other animals—it is to be "lightly valued." He was not the only influential theologian who associated reason with human nature. Ambrose identified animals with human passions, and even interpreted the first book of Genesis as a testimony to how human beings should control their passions, and how the mind is superior to those passions.[24] Augustine's later interpretation of Genesis showed a similar tendency to see human control over passions as being represented in the Genesis text that speaks of the relationship between human beings and other animals. Here, too, there is a reiteration of his earlier thought that human beings resemble God only insofar as they have reason and understanding.[25] Though he allowed for the possibility that the woman had the powers of reasoning, in her sexuality she remains subject to the man, and such impulses had to come under the control of the mind's reasoning powers. Inasmuch as women were perceived to be closer to animals, women were "made for man."[26]

Augustine did not just focus on mental activity in speaking about the distinctive aspects of human life. He also understood God through metaphors drawn from human mental activity, such as choosing, willing, remembering, and understanding. As Janet Soskice remarks, "Augustine constantly privileged mind over body, sometimes identifying the self with mind alone, and sometimes speaking of the mind as *using* the body" (emphasis in the original).[27] Although Augustine rejects the idea around at his time that the woman is simply the symbolic marker for the body, and that the man is the symbolic marker for the mind, the kind of mental knowledge permitted for women is practical *scientia*, whereas that for men is of a higher order, *sapientia*, wisdom.[28]

Here it is worth defining more clearly how intellectual and cultural history have developed in this particular case. Is it valid—or even justifiable, in other words—to look back at Augustine for precedents to our contemporary positions? Given Augustine's elevation of the mind, it is hardly surprising that he has been represented as one of the pillars of the Western metaphysical tradition that led to Cartesian subjectivity and was then translated into the nihilism of Nietzsche, Heidegger, and their followers. In his influential book *Sources of Self: The Making of the Modern Identity*, Charles Taylor seems to endorse this approach to cultural history, and thus he places Augustine firmly between Plato and Descartes. Here he argues that the Christian distinction between flesh and spirit came to be understood through Plato's distinction between bodily and nonbodily forms, understood in terms of inner spirit and outer bodily sense.[29] He believes that Augustine shifted knowledge of God from outer experiences to those internal to the human mind. Thus, in what has sometimes been called the *proto-cogito*, Augustine claims that existence is linked with the possibility of deception, and thus establishes the importance of the self.[30]

Taylor's inclusion of Augustine in an intellectual history from Plato to Descartes is criticized by Michael Hanby, who believes that the main nihilistic influence on Descartes is not so much Augustine as a Stoic philosophy of the will that Augustine rejected in the name of Christ and the Trinity.[31] It seems to me that Hanby is correct to resist the idea that modernity arises out of a singular event, or that it can be reduced to a single corruption. He also believes that Augustine's focus on doxology means that he cannot be characterized as "proto-Cartesian." But to separate Augustine from the rest of cultural history may be going too far in the other direction. What is more important, perhaps, is a comparison of the *function* of arguments in different philosophies, rather than coming to firm conclusions about precursors in a direct evolutionary lineage of ideas. It seems to me that Augustine *did* ground his thinking in a strong doctrine of creation, a doxological appreciation of the importance of worship in Christian life, and an understanding of God in mystical terms. All this *qualified* his focus on human mental activity. However, it can hardly be denied that he influenced the association of mental activity with human flourishing, and therefore his influence in subsequent generations was profound, even if it would be false to conclude that he was the only thinker in this vein, or that he was directly responsible for Descartes's position. In this we can envisage such cultural history as comprising a *meshwork* of ideas that gradually develops over time, rather than a simple linear pattern of cultural inheritance.

Once belief in God was no longer convincing, those who adhered to its secular residue still hoped for salvation through human mental aspirations. Expressions of transhumanity as they emerge in the Western context are therefore secular versions of very ancient theological and philosophical debates—but now stripped bare of any explicit theological reference markers. The sources of influence on such ideas are likely to be complex rather than linear, but the pattern of thinking that assumes mental activity is the prime source of happiness, along with a failure to take bodily nature as a good in itself, shows up once again in this modern philosophy. Behind this we find an echo of Plato's thought that ethical self-sufficiency arises from a self-sufficient intellect, with bodily appetites pushed into the background. As Martha Nussbaum has pointed out, Aristotelian thought pointed in another direction, namely toward a view "that permits us to see our neediness vis-à-vis the world as not inimical to, but at the very heart of, our ethical value."[32] Aristotle argues that the disconnection of human lives from the functioning of living beings in general was mistaken.

It also seems reasonable to suggest that those theologians who will find disembodied aspirations of transhumanism and its variants the most attractive will be those who adhere to metaphors of God filtered through mental activity and imagery, rather than bodily nature. Human image bearing then becomes connected to the image of God by expressing a form of creative superintelligence. Humans share in this intelligence by becoming cocreators with God. Conversely, those theologians who have been influenced by, for example, feminist thinking or ecotheology are more likely to object, given the focus of these theologies on interconnectedness and bodily nature, alongside appropriate recognition of the differences between men, women, and other animals.

For these kinds of thinkers, and I count myself as broadly belonging among them, transhuman philosophy of the type peddled by Bostrom fails not just because it seems to promote disconnection within the self (mind and body), while offering a materialistic atheism, but also because it promotes disconnection between selves. Social goods seem to be added as an afterthought, and only when viewed as an aspect of the good for the particular individual. Its language of human development is univocal, protected by a veil of scientific respectability and feeding off the real needs and desires of those who are suffering, in order to project futures that are barely recognized as reasonable by those medical practitioners involved.[33] Yet the subtle influence of such projections on the public acceptability of such technologies and therefore their likely incorporation into societal goods can hardly be denied.

Alternative Models of Human Flourishing

To address the real challenge of transhumanism and its vision for the future, those theologians who find themselves uneasy with its trajectory do so because of their adherence to alternative ways of viewing what human flourishing might be like. Instead of an exclusive emphasis on the mental powers of willing, choosing, and understanding, human futures need to include more bodily metaphors of gestating, relating, and nurturing. Sexual difference is then included along with other differences, such as that between humanity and other animals, so that it is a difference in degree rather than an absolute one. An emphasis on treating all creatures as "Thou" instead of "It," to use Martin Buber's terminology, changes the ethos of human aspiration from one that is driven by technological achievement to one that is filtered through human goods, worked out in collaboration and in consultation with others. A shift toward relationship is a reminder that life that is received as a gift includes the giftedness of others in relation to human beings. Although not exclusively a Christian concept, the notion of gift and the welcome of the other *as other* counteracts the more hubristic tendency for control over uncertain futures that is woven into transhumanism.[34] If other creatures are viewed as gifts, animals will then no longer be used as a means to achieve narrow human ends, and the fate of other peoples as well as particular elite cultures are more likely to come into view.

In this context, one of the buried ethical problems with transhumanism is the health injustice that it seems to promote, the disproportionate spending on what might be termed exotic science, even while claiming to be an aspiration for the majority of people, because such an aspiration is out of touch with even the most simplistic concrete models of economics and development. If those living in the world's poorest regions were to be given access to transhuman technology, the possibilities of exploitation and lack of regulation would be rife. Similar worries arise, for example, in the very real case of stem cell research. At the moment stem cell research is not a feature of the research landscape of the world's poorest regions. But if it spreads to these regions, where the political and policy infrastructures for its appropriate regulation are not in place, the possible opportunities for its exploitation are legion.[35]

In reaching for control of the human person and its future, transhumanism entirely misses the possibility that human beings are complex creatures who resist reduction to functional mental units. In the wake of postmodern culture theologians have become increasingly drawn to those forms of theology that resist spelling out in detail what God is like, and what human beings are like. The problem with transhumanism is that it seems to remove any sense of mystery—any admission of ignorance other than the uncertainty of not knowing which scenario will play out in future human projections. The scenario that something else entirely might dawn in human history is not even considered, except inasmuch as that the new is strictly wedded to technological invention. I am not suggesting by this that all technology should be resisted, but rather the use of a particular transhuman futurist project that filters the direction of that technology.

The kind of flourishing projected by transhumanism is one of perfectionism molded by a particular cybercultural set of values and concerns. If such technology were to become commonplace, those choosing not to take up such opportunities might be considered irresponsible. A similar pressure already exists on families who choose not to undertake prenatal tests for certain genetic diseases, for example.[36] The transhuman project is eugenic insofar as it is a deliberate strategy for affirming and maintaining indefinitely only some forms of human life. The idea of solidarity prominent in Roman Catholic social teaching, based on a shared human condition, is no longer tenable in a transhuman world, for the human itself is now being transformed away from its roots in shared creaturely being. In the encyclical *Caritas in veritate*, Pope Benedict XVI has argued that materialistic and mechanistic understandings of human life undermine a sense of human dignity, whereby he means that life is a mystery to be respected. This mechanistic understanding is, for him, a "culture of death" in such a way that conscience is dulled and the interior life is reduced to neurology.[37] The goals of transhumanism extend far beyond the scenarios that Pope Benedict seems to have appreciated in this encyclical. His comments were focused on what is currently possible in the manipulation of embryos and end-of-life technologies. If fears and anxieties and other forms of suffering are engineered out of the human condition in the manner advocated by transhumanism, then any residue of sensitivity to the spiritual dimension is likely to be lost.

Concluding Remarks: Taking Leave of the Animal

I have argued in this chapter that whereas the kind of perfectionism offered through transhumanism of the variety proposed by Nick Bostrom might appeal in an age growing accustomed to new and exotic forms of technology, inasmuch as it distances the human from its creaturely bearings, it fails to provide an adequate account of human flourishing. By attempting to control particular contingent problems of the human condition, it inadvertently commits an error that is ancient in its roots: attempting to find succor by distancing the human from its material, creaturely, animal origins. Ironically, perhaps, such hubristic attempts to control also bring risks that are recognized by its protagonists. However, the assumption that legal restraint will be sufficient does not adequately address the social dimension of these technologies. The tendency for theologians to distance human flourishing from that of other creatures and other animals in particular is evident in the thought of Augustine of Hippo onward. However, Augustine's strong focus on belief in creation and the Trinity offset much of this tendency.

In the contemporary context, where evolution by natural selection has elbowed out stronger beliefs in the fixity of the cosmos, the remnant reminiscent of Augustinian thinking tends to be read through a modern lens. This means that a strong sense of human solidarity with other animals has gone, making way for tolerance or even affirmation of transhuman philosophies. Such a tendency also brings other dangers, because not only might we be inclined to treat other animals as means through which to fulfill transhuman projects, but the focus is also away from the concerns of other human beings living in areas where even the most basic human needs are not met.

To commit the fallacy of inevitability is to fail to see transhumanism as a *human* technological project, and one that is shaped by human society. It is a fallacy in two senses. First, it is a fallacy in the sense that technological change is viewed as having a momentum of its own that cannot be changed or adjusted. Those committed to this philosophy create the impression that such changes are now going to happen anyway, so any ethical reflection must be about what to do with such developments. But this forgets the fact that human beings are agents of their own destiny, and thus it seems akin to fatalism.

Second, such a belief shapes moral discourse in that it gives up on questioning the possibility that power may be exerted in particular ways to arrive at such a scenario. Moral reflection is thin insofar as it is about what the goods might be of a given social and political change, rather than challenging whether such changes are desirable or not. I have tried to argue in this chapter that such changes are in many respects far from desirable inasmuch as they detach human flourishing from other creatures and thus reinforce a false sense of human superiority. Further, to be more humane, scenarios about human becoming need to recognize the animal roots of human beings and flourishing, rather than vainly attempt to distance human lives from these roots.

Notes

Celia Deane-Drummond presented a modified version of this chapter as a lecture titled "Taking Leave of the Animal: Transhumanity as Transanimality" at the Critical Annual Studies Conference, organized by Stephen Clark, at Liverpool University, Liverpool, April 23, 2010. She thanks the organizers for the invitation and the participants who gave her valuable feedback.

1. By trajectory I mean in a primary sense a historical process of intellectual descent. However, I also mean that which pushes toward the future in a particular way as an intellectual concept that gathers momentum over time, even if, as in this particular case, it is not acknowledged. A linear trajectory implies a straight line, but trajectory as such should not necessarily imply this. Cultural evolution might be better conceived as a *meshwork* of ideas, rather than a straight line in a manner a little analogous to biological evolution, though the mechanisms involved are distinct.

2. Harris, *Enhancing Evolution*, 8.

3. Ibid., 11.

4. Ibid., 13.

5. The idea of controlling our own evolution has a pedigree that dates back to eugenics and the dreams of geneticists in the middle of the last century, such as H. J. Muller. For him the worry was that unless steps were taken to actively intervene in genetics, then we would turn into monsters. This was because if modern medicine permitted those with diseases to survive, then the processes of natural selection could no longer weed out the weakest members of society. See Muller, "Guidance of Human Evolution." Of course, the prospect that genetic manipulation might prove to be a vehicle of artificial evolution is actually

unrealistic, even by the simplest equations of population genetics, unless all carriers of disease are treated similarly. Further, given the history of eugenics, biologists are more often than not reluctant to make any bold claims for social and political change. Harris seems to ignore this aspect entirely in his recommendations. For further discussion of the influence of eugenics, see Deane-Drummond, *Genetics and Christian Ethics*, 55–75.

6. For a summary of his work on risk, see, e.g., Bostrom and Ćirković, *Global Catastrophic Risks*.

7. Nick Bostrom comments that "it is important to attempt (as best we can) to distinguish futuristic scenarios put forward for their symbolic significance or entertainment value from speculations that are meant to be evaluated on the basis of literal plausibility. Only the latter form of 'realistic' futuristic thought will be considered in this paper." See Bostrom, "Future of Humanity," also published in Olsen, Selinger, and Riis, *New Waves in Philosophy*, 2. Such an approach effectively wipes out cultural history in one fell swoop, and in the manner akin to his Oxford colleague Richard Dawkins, he dismisses religion as in the same category with science fiction. Like Dawkins, he is trying to convince his readers that his speculations are based or grounded in hard science.

8. Olsen, Selinger, and Riis, *New Waves*, 5.

9. Harris uses a similar argument to argue his case for transhumanism in *Enhancing Evolution*, 12–13.

10. Bostrom, "Future of Humanity," 16. He discusses a swath of other possible methods of cognitive enhancements, some in use, and some more speculative; see Bostrom and Sandberg, "Cognitive Enhancement."

11. It is worth noting that Bostrom has worked with physicists and cosmologists, and his understanding that this is possible according to physical laws seems to be broadly correct. See, e.g., Bostrom and Ćirković, *Global Catastrophic Risks*.

12. The way Bostrom is using "posthumanity" is different from the way the term is often used in cultural studies. For Bostrom, posthumanity means a human condition where human capacities are enhanced through scientific means. It is therefore dependent on the Enlightenment mentality that elevates the human. In cultural studies, however, the term "posthuman" more often than not seems to refer to an unsettling of assumptions about the human, perhaps through the image of the Cyborg, in a manner that has some kinship with postmodern theory. It can therefore be used in critical animal studies, an emerging field that explores in a critical way current relationships between human beings and other animals. Whether Bostrom is justified in using the term "posthuman" in this way is outside the scope of this chapter.

13. See, e.g., Bostrom and Sandberg, "Cognitive Enhancement," 17–18.

14. Boulle, *La Planet de Singes*; Wells, *Island of Dr Moreau*. Also see Brin, *Uplift War*, the third volume in Brin's *The Uplift Saga*.

15. As this chapter goes to press, Richard Twine's book *Animals as Biotechnology* has been brought to my attention. This book reflects the work of a sociologist who is particularly concerned to raise the social issues connection with animal

biotechnologies. It also aims to challenge the complacent attitude toward the way humans treat other animals.

16. Animal rights terminology may put animals on the agenda, but, rather like human rights language, it tends to be divisive and worked out amid conflicts of rights interests. Andrew Linzey, for example, is hostile toward all animal biotechnology, describing genetic engineering of animals as a form of animal slavery. Linzey, *Animal Theology*. Given the growth in animal biotechnology—e.g., as outlined by Rehbinder et al., *Pharming*—I find it somewhat astonishing that he has not considered this topic at all in his most recent book on animal suffering. Cf. Linzey, *Why Animal Suffering Matters*. My own preference would be to develop a virtue approach to animal ethics that would be permissible with respect to some forms of technology, but not others; cf. Deane-Drummond, *Ethics of Nature*, 54–110.

17. Holland and Johnson, "Introduction," in *Animal Biotechnology and Ethics*, 7.

18. Once the idea of inevitability is accepted, the only form of control seems to be legal restriction. See Burkhardt, "Inevitability of Animal Biotechnology?" 114–32.

19. Thompson, "Biotechnology Policy," 262.

20. The beginning of such a task is discussed by Deane-Drummond and Clough, *Creaturely Theology*, final section.

21. See more discussion of virtues given by Deane-Drummond, "Future Perfect?"

22. Augustine, *On the Literal Interpretation of Genesis*, chap. 16:59, p. 186.

23. Ibid., chap. 16:60, p. 186.

24. Ambrose, *Paradise*, 11, 51–52.

25. As given by Saint Augustine, *Confessions*, book XIII, p. 34.

26. According to Augustine, the only sense in which woman is made for man is through the possibility of physical reproduction. Hence, he states that "in the physical sense, woman has been made for man. In her mind, and her natural intelligence, she has a nature the equal of man's, but in sex she is physically subject to him"; ibid., 34. Augustine's recognition of woman's equal intelligence makes Augustine a "proto-feminist," according to Soskice, *Kindness of God*, 43.

27. Ibid., 133.

28. Ibid., 135–36.

29. Taylor, *Sources of Self*, 127.

30. This term *proto-cogito* follows the terminology of Descartes, who was later to make the claim *cogito esse*—i.e., I think, therefore I am.

31. Hanby, *Augustine and Modernity*, 135. It strikes me that Hanby does not take sufficiently into account the way that Taylor at least attempts to qualify his ideas, at least in places, by showing up the novelty of Descartes compared with Augustine. He also allows for the fact that Augustine retains a Platonic notion of order in the cosmos as a good that further qualifies his suggestion that Augustine is an originator of the turn inward to the self. Cf. Taylor, *Sources*, 129, 143. There are clearly overlapping fields of understanding here, though how far he is correct to identify a lineage is difficult to judge.

32. Nussbaum, *Fragility of Goodness*, 264.

33. At a colloquium that I organized in 2005 in order to prepare for the book published in 2006 titled *Future Perfect?* the medical scientists who took part found discussions of transhumanism and posthumanism difficult to comprehend or connect with their ordinary working life.

34. This is pointed out by Sandel, *Case against Perfection*, 85–100. By this he means the belief that life is received, rather than originated through deliberate choice. The concept of life as a gift from a divine source is shared by other religious traditions, but Sandel wants to remove any reference to theism. He also seems to conflate the idea of gift with giftedness, which amounts to a hierarchical rating of some individuals over others through a special natural talent or ability. Theologians who object to new reproductive technologies have sometimes based their arguments around gift versus choice. However, the idea that any sort of choice might reduce the acceptance of a resulting child as a gift seems to me to be a weak argument given the current level of uncertainty associated with all reproductive technologies. What needs to be resisted is the illusion that children can be chosen for specific characteristics. Bostrom and others believe that there will come a time when this is no longer illusory, and enhancements become more or less guaranteed. This scenario is, of course, highly speculative. Here we might challenge the wisdom of parents and others in making such choices for the genuine societal good of future generations.

35. This issue was raised by those participants from the poorest regions of the world at a World Council of Churches Consultation on Stem Cells, Volos Theological Academy, November 8–12, 2009.

36. See Deane-Drummond, *Genetics and Christian Ethics*, 84–86.

37. Benedict XVI, *Caritas in Veritate*, paragraphs 75–76.

References

Ambrose. *Paradise*, translated by Andrew Louth in collaboration with Marco Conti. In *Ancient Christian Commentary on Scripture, Old Testament, Genesis 1–11*. London: Fitzroy Dearborn Publishers, 2001.

Augustine. *Confessions*, translated by R. S. Pine-Coffin. London: Penguin Books, 1961.

Augustine. *On the Literal Interpretation of Genesis: An Unfinished Book*, translated by Roland J. Teske. In *The Fathers of the Church. A New Translation*. Washington, DC: Catholic University of America Press, 1991.

Bostrom, Nick. "The Future of Humanity." Available at www.nickbostrom.com.

Bostrom, Nick, and Milan M. Ćirković. *Global Catastrophic Risks*. Oxford: Oxford University Press, 2008.

Bostrom, Nick, and Anders Sandberg. "Cognitive Enhancement: Methods, Ethics, Regulatory Challenges." *Science and Engineering Ethics* 15, no. 3 (2009): 311–41.

Boulle, P. *La Planet de Singes*. Paris: Hachette, 1963.

Brin, David. *The Uplift War*. New York: Bantam, 1987.

Burkhardt, Jeffrey. "The Inevitability of Animal Biotechnology? Ethics and the Scientific Attitude." in *Animal Biotechnology and Ethics*, edited by Alan Holland and Alan Johnson. London: Routledge, 1998, 113–32.

Deane-Drummond, Celia. *The Ethics of Nature*. Oxford: Blackwell/Wiley, 2004.

———. *Genetics and Christian Ethics*. Cambridge: Cambridge University Press, 2006.

———. "Future Perfect: God, the Transhuman Future, and the Quest for Immortality." in *Future Perfect?: God, Medicine and Human Identity*, 2nd ed., edited by Celia Deane-Drummond and Peter Manley Scott. London: Continuum, 2010.

Deane-Drummond, Celia, and David Clough, eds. *Creaturely Theology: On God, Humans and Other Animals*. London: SCM Press, 2009.

Hanby, M. *Augustine and Modernity*. London: Routledge, 2003.

Harris, John. *Enhancing Evolution: The Ethical Case for Making Better People*. Princeton, NJ: Princeton University Press, 2007.

Holland, Alan, and Alan Johnson, eds. *Animal Biotechnology and Ethics*. London: Routledge, 1998.

Linzey, Andrew. *Animal Theology*. London: SPCK, 1994.

———. *Why Animal Suffering Matters: Philosophy, Theology and Practical Ethics*. Oxford: Oxford University Press, 2009.

Muller, H. J. "The Guidance of Human Evolution." *Perspectives in Biology and Medicine* 3 (1959): 1–43.

Nussbaum, Martha. *The Fragility of Goodness: Luck and Ethics in Greek Tragedy and Philosophy*, 2nd ed. Cambridge: Cambridge University Press, 2001.

Olsen, Jan-Kyrre Berg, Evan Selinger, and Søren Riis, eds. *New Waves in Philosophy and Technology*. New York: Palgrave Macmillan, 2009.

Pope Benedict XVI. *Caritas in veritate*. Vatican City: The Holy See, 2009.

Rehbinder, E., M. Engelhard, K. Hagen, R. B. Jorgensen, R. Pardo-Avellaneda, A. Schnieke, and F. Thiele. *Pharming: Promises and Risks of Biopharmaceuticals Derived from Genetically Modified Plants and Animals*. Berlin: Springer-Verlag, 2009.

Sandel, Michael. *The Case against Perfection: Ethics in an Age of Genetic Engineering*. Cambridge, MA: Belknap Press of Harvard University Press, 2007.

Soskice, Janet. *The Kindness of God: Metaphor, Gender, and Religious Language*. Oxford: Oxford University Press, 2007.

Taylor, Charles. *Sources of Self: The Making of the Modern Identity*. Cambridge: Cambridge University Press, 1989.

Thompson, Paul B. *Biotechnology Policy: Four Ethical Problems and Three Political Solutions*. College Station, TX: Texas A&M University, 1996.

Twine, Richard. *Animals as Biotechnology: Ethics, Sustainability and Critical Animal Studies*. London: Earthscan, 2010.

Wells, H. G. *The Island of Dr Moreau*. New Orleans: Heinemann, 1896.

Chapter Nine

Chasing Methuselah

Transhumanism and Christian *Theosis* in
Critical Perspective

TODD T. W. DALY

On Monday, August 4, 1997, Madame Jeanne Calment died at the age
of 122 years as the longest-lived person in modern history. Before
her death she had become a local celebrity in her hometown of Arles,
France. She took up fencing at the age of 85 and was still riding her bicycle at
100. She was fond of both chocolate and cigarettes, and only reluctantly gave
up the latter two years before her death, when she became unable to light
cigarettes on her own. Though she claimed that the secrets to her longevity
were port wine and olive oil, few who might choose to follow her "regimen"
could hope to replicate her results. Indeed, though the chances of reaching
the upper biological limit of 120 years are extremely remote, the last century
has witnessed a dramatic increase in life expectancy, from about 50 years in
1900 to nearly 80 in 2000.[1] These unprecedented gains in life expectancy can
be attributed primarily to medical breakthroughs, ranging from the effective treatment of acute illnesses and diseases like tuberculosis and smallpox
and the reduction of the infant mortality rate to improvements in sanitary
conditions.

Nevertheless, for many the prospect of greatly extended—if not indefinite—healthy longevity is enormously attractive. Thomas Nagle once com-
mented that given the choice between living another week or dying in five
minutes, he would always choose to live another week, concluding through
mathematical induction that he would be happy to live forever.[2] With the
promise of technology, we may no longer need to rely on such hackneyed
formulas as port wine and olive oil for longevity. We thus find ourselves in
the predicament described in Aeschylus's *Prometheus Bound*. Having stolen
fire from Zeus and given it to human beings, Prometheus declares to the
daughters of Oceanos that he has given human beings something to prevent
them from "brooding over death," the inescapability of finitude, by lodging
"blind hopes" in their hearts.[3] Yet, with fire or *techné*, humans now had the
ability to forestall death. This combination of the certainty of death and the

blind hope for averting its arrival are two primary forces that underwrite contemporary medical practice and the search for longer, healthier lives.[4] However, most in the scientific community agree that surpassing the biological barrier will require altering the aging process itself. Recent attempts to do just this have shown some success in the laboratory.

Antiaging Medicine: From Legend to Laboratory

Researchers have been able to slow the aging process of multicellular organisms and animals in the laboratory with techniques like selective breeding, dietary restrictions, and genetic manipulation. The healthy life span of mice has been extended by 70 percent by utilizing a combination of genetic alterations and dietary or caloric restrictions.[5] Indeed, one of the most promising avenues of aging research involves the link between fasting and aging. The hope is to manufacture a pill that mimics the changes of genetic manipulation, which would allow us to enjoy the benefits of fasting without any change or reduction in food intake. Other researchers have extended the life span of the nematode worm sevenfold by altering a single gene.[6]

Breakthroughs like these are beginning to alter our perception of aging. The researchers Guarente and Kenyon observe: "When single genes are changed, animals that should be old stay young. In humans these old mutants would be analogous to a ninety year old who looks and feels forty-five. On this basis we begin to think of ageing as a disease that can be cured, or at least postponed."[7] It is significant that these extensions are marked by health and vitality, which assuages fears that we might simply be prolonging the length of old age and its attendant afflictions. The indisputable goal involves extending the *healthy* life span and avoiding a prolonged decline, an enormously attractive prospect in a culture obsessed with youth and morbidly fearful of death. Closely related is the hope that aging attenuation may dramatically shorten the period of decline before death, a period that has been steadily increasing due to constant developments in technology.

For a growing number of researchers and scientists, the ultimate enemy is not death but the aging process itself.[8] The prospect of having an additional thirty to fifty years of health to pursue innumerable athletic, artistic, and intellectual projects is an alluring thought. Though historically aging has not been considered a disease, it is increasingly being viewed as a treatable disorder and thus as amenable to clinical therapy. Though not all scientists believe that humans ought to understand the human aging process for the explicit purpose of manipulating it, the project of extending life via aging attenuation is now garnering more mainstream medical support.[9]

Indeed, transhumanist philosophy actively encourages the relatively recent forays into understanding the human aging process, known broadly as biogerontology, in hopes that one day aging might prove susceptible to technological intervention. Transhumanism is a movement comprising philosophers and scientists and others devoted to using all forms of technology to pursue the goal of eliminating death and all forms of suffering endemic to embodied existence. Though the desire for indefinite longevity resonates with many, transhumanist philosophy has seized upon this general sentiment and has assigned it a place of preeminence in the desire to transcend current human bodily limitations and obstacles posed by the cumbersome and wasteful evolutionary process. More breathtaking vistas of transhuman life envision an earthly immortality rid of the body altogether. Though some transhumanists, like Ray Kurzweil, routinely speak of the promise of nanobots, digital digestion, programmable blood, and nonbiological brains en route to digitizing and uploading the mind to more powerful computers, others like the former Cambridge geneticist Aubrey de Grey have formed research companies like the Methuselah Foundation, which focus on finding a "cure" for aging by rendering senescence (cellular aging) negligible, and predict life spans of several millennia as early as 2025.[10] The Methuselah Foundation, which was named after the Old Testament figure in the Book of Genesis (5:27) who lived nearly a millennium, is one among several new organizations devoted to slowing the human aging process, such as Elixir Pharmaceuticals, Juvenon, Biomarker Pharmaceuticals, and Centagenetix.[11]

The Transhumanist Vision

The two core beliefs driving the transhumanist agenda are that human existence is unnecessarily held captive to the death, decay, and disease inherent in the evolutionary process and that the application of a host of "smarter" technologies—including prosthetics, genetic engineering, pharmacology, molecular nanocomputing, and artificial intelligence—will enable us to mitigate and eventually eliminate the effects of aging and disease altogether, at which point we will move into the *post*human realm. It is little wonder, then, that some transhumanists describe themselves as the "New Prometheans," who grasp at transcendence via the torch of technology, which illuminates the new knowledge whereby humans may one day banish the limitations inherent in embodiment.[12] The transhumanists collectively grate against any suggestion, however, that these are "blind hopes," as Prometheus declared, and thus summarily dismiss any objections to their visions of longevity. Indeed, the transhumanists celebrate the fact that the search for the fountain of youth or the creation of the *elixir vitae* has moved from legend to laboratory.

Many technological hurdles remain, and transhumanists typically underestimate their significance. Yet the potential effects of even modestly extended life spans cut across all aspects of human life—from economic stability and the supportability of an increasingly aging population, to issues of intragenerational equity, to environmental and ecosystem stability. The idea of extending life beyond current biological limits also raises interesting moral questions that are often suppressed by the collective enthusiasm and utopian-like prognostications of many transhumanists. Moreover, those who question the role technology should play in human flourishing are typically charged with having an irrational sense of dread and labeled "bio-Luddites," who are described as those "who wish to abandon human progress for a perpetual present."[13]

Any hesitations expressed on religious grounds elicit similar responses. Because, for instance, the Christian faith speaks of life after death based on the resurrection of Jesus Christ from the dead, the transhumanists charge Christians with being largely unconcerned about the length of one's life, or worse as people who happily accept death. One of transhumanism's apologists, Simon Young, has coined the term "thanatosia" for just such a position (from the Greek word for death, *thanatos*).[14] The transhumanists often assume that the Christian faith has no vested interest in greatly extended healthy lives, and thus they point for instance to the statement of the apostle Paul: "To live is Christ and to die is gain" (Phil. 1:21). But such transhumanist criticisms rest at best on a rather thin description of the Christian faith, and at worst on an outright caricature of it. For the view that our bodies may be reformed to enhance the possibilities of greater longevity is not entirely antithetical to the Christian faith. Indeed, it is worth noting that one of the figureheads at the birth of modern medicine, Francis Bacon (1561–1626), asserted that prolongevity was the most noble goal of medicine and posed little difficulties for Christians making their way toward Heaven.[15] He believed that increasing control over the created order was *the* means by which humanity might regain the bodily immortality that Adam and Eve forfeited in the Garden of Eden.[16] Bacon drew upon the imagery of a return to Eden in his own call for the exploration of the mechanisms involved in human aging, and he attempted to situate (with some difficulty) the pursuit of greater longevity within the Christian narrative inscribed by the crucifixion, death, resurrection, and ascension of Jesus Christ, which culminates in the redeemed creation living in glorified, resurrection bodies in God's presence.

Indeed, the belief that one might put on something of the incorruptible body in a return to Eden is rooted deep in the Christian tradition, and intimately related to what is commonly known as *theosis*. The concept of *theosis*—becoming divine or Godlike—finds its roots in Holy Scripture, and it has continued as one of several metaphors for salvation in the catholic (universal) church, from church fathers like Irenaeus, Clement of Alexandria, Athanasius, and Gregory of Nyssa, to later theologians like Thomas Aquinas, Martin Luther, and John Wesley.[17] Although the metaphysical aspects of *theosis* might be articulated with the concept of participation (*methexis*) in God (2 Pt 1:4) or other metaphors present in the Christian tradition, the ethical dimension of *theosis* has entailed the practice of several disciplines that have viewed the body as both *integral to* and the *beneficiary of* character formation. One of the benefits of a disciplined life was thought to be greater longevity through the slowing of human aging.

As we shall see, Saint Athanasius of Alexandria (c. 293–373 CE) asserted that human aging could be considerably attenuated and the human life span could thus be significantly extended, a process he described as a return to prelapsarian, or pre-Fall, Eden. But the achievement of this heightened longevity involved the ascetic discipline of bodily fasting to refine one's soul—a discipline epitomized by the desert ascetic Saint Antony (c. 251–356)—whereby one could attain the prelapsarian state of Adam in the Garden of Eden. Therefore, it is worth exploring Athanasius's account of a return to Adamic life in the garden. Any Christian consideration of life extension, however, must be informed by the last Adam, Jesus Christ. For this, I draw on the Christology of Karl Barth, speaking in particular of the body and its relationship to the soul, including attitudes concerning our perceived life span. Before turning to Barth's consideration of the body–soul relationship as revealed in Jesus Christ, I examine Athanasius's understanding of longevity with regard to the body and soul.

Athanasius on Remaking the Body: Adam Again

In *On the Incarnation* Athanasius writes that Adam's original state in the Garden of Eden reflected the body and soul in perfect order: The soul was in submission to God, and the body was in perfect submission to the soul. Though Adam's body was always tending toward decay, his soul was thought to offer some attenuation to human aging, as long as his soul was in submission to God. When Adam sinned, however, by turning his attention away from God to other material things, his body and soul were effectively thrown into disorder and dissolution—his body began to rule his soul—thereby bringing

God's pronouncement of death and hastening the decaying process inherent in Adam's body. It is this condition, says Athanasius, that the incarnate Word, Jesus Christ, came to rectify.

Although Athanasius speaks of Christ's death as a ransom or satisfaction of debt, his primary emphasis is on *theosis*, Christ's restoration of the divine image in us.[18] Based in part on 2 Peter 1:4, which speaks of our participation in the divine nature, Athanasius repeats an already well-known "formula," that Christ "was made man that we might be made God," asserting that part of this deification is *bodily* in nature.[19] Thus, though Athanasius admittedly describes the Fall in Platonic terms as having been occasioned by inordinate attention to material things, the way back to Paradise begins by attending to the body.

The paradigmatic figure for *theosis* is the desert ascetic Saint Antony, who displays powers over disease, demons, and seemingly death itself. But Athanasius is most impressed by Antony's ability to restore the proper order of body and soul. By fasting, Athanasius asserts, Antony was able to reorder the body and soul, restoring the soul as the rightful leader of the body, and thereby regaining some of that bodily integrity and resistance to aging that were originally found in the Garden of Eden. Indeed, fasting as such becomes more significant given that several church fathers spoke of Adam and Eve's sin in terms of gluttony. But Athanasius records that through fasting and prayer, Saint Antony lived to the age of 105 years, many of them in the harsh conditions of the North African desert. In the early church there is ample evidence of the belief that the body's decay could be effectively slowed down by fasting, thereby "putting on a little of that incorruption" enjoyed by Adam in the garden. Athanasius, however, also realized that any discussion of a return to Paradise must be balanced by the promise of the future bodily resurrection, reminding us that only Christ can clothe us with immortality.

Athanasius makes it clear that the goal of fasting is not primarily to attain a longer life but to bring the soul into submission to God, and the body into submission to the soul. Among the Desert Fathers, fasting was recognized as a crucial first step in reordering one's body and soul. Only after one had effectively "quieted" the impulses of one's body could one most effectively begin to till the hardened soil of one's heart and will. Though we might view such ascetic endeavors as unnecessarily harsh, restrictive, or isolating, Douglas Burton-Christie observes that "the *telos* [purpose] of the monks' life in the desert was freedom: freedom from anxiety about the future; freedom from the tyranny of haunting memories of the past; freedom from an attachment to the ego which precluded intimacy with others and with God. They hoped also that this freedom would express itself in a positive sense:

freedom to love others; freedom to enjoy the presence of God; freedom to live in the innocence of a new paradise."[20] In Athanasius, the body is heavily implicated in the transformation of one's soul. Thus, though Athanasius recognized that slowing aging was possible, it was never the primary goal but was rather *subsumed* under the moral project of the transformation of one's soul. Hence the body was far from neutral. Bodily life is not simply collapsed under the weight of the spirit or the autonomous will, but, as Oliver O'Donovan has explained, "bodily life . . . is given to *sustain* spiritual life, and in turn to be *renewed* by it."[21]

The Desert Fathers sought to regain the condition of Adam before the Fall, a pathway that began with fasting to restore the soul in submission to God as the rightful ruler of one's body. In acknowledging that the Desert Fathers construed the pathway to transformation as an attempt to return to Paradise by regaining the state of the first Adam, a Christian understanding of human aging and embodiment requires that we say something in light of the coming of the second Adam, the Incarnation of the Word, Jesus Christ.

Adam Again: The Real Man Jesus According to Karl Barth

Barth's account of human nature and thriving is relentlessly Christological. For Barth, we cannot possibly know what it means to be human apart from "the nature of man as it confronts us in the person of Jesus."[22] Human nature is not discerned in advance from science, philosophy, or the social sciences. Rather, we learn what it means to be human in the history of a particular individual in whom human nature—and nature itself—is vindicated, restored, and exalted. For, as T. F. Torrance has noted, the Incarnation is not God *in* a human being, but God *as* a human.[23] In particular, Barth's reflections on the nature of the body–soul relationship based on the real man Jesus offer unique insights on our finitude and the current disorder of body and soul. Because Barth was wary of the reductionist anthropology of scientific materialism on the one hand and the uncritical appropriation of Greek dualism on the other, he put forward what has been termed a "dynamic anthropology," or a "dialectical–dialogical" approach, with respect to the body and soul.[24]

To understand the relationship between body and soul, we must look to the one true man, Jesus, who provides the ontological determination of what it means to be human. Barth asserts that the man Jesus is the one whole man, "embodied soul and besouled body," by whom we judge what it means to have a soul and a body.[25] Unlike fallen humanity, however, in Jesus there is no war or "ascetic conflict" between the body and the soul. The Spirit of God resting on the man Jesus, asserts Barth, renders asceticism "superfluous."[26] The body is neither the conqueror nor enemy of the soul; nor does the soul masquerade as the enemy or conqueror of the body. To the contrary, says Barth, Jesus is the picture of peace "between these two moments of human existence."[27] He continues:

> Jesus spoke and acted and suffered in obedience and omnipotence in and not without His body, so that He was also wholly this body. Yet His action and passion are first, *a parte potiori* [from the preferable part], those of His soul, and in that way and on that basis of His body. His body is used and governed by Him for the purpose of a specific and conscious speech and action and suffering. It serves Him in the execution of His purpose. It is impregnated with soul, . . . a soul filled by the needs and desires of His bodily life. This is the distinction and inequality to be noted within the oneness and the wholeness. The fulfilment, the willing and the execution and therefore the true movement of his body occurs from above downwards, from the soul to body and not *vice versa*.[28]

Unlike Jesus, however, we allow our body and soul to "go their separate ways," and thus allow the drives of the body to have undue influence on the soul, to the extent that we desire and will the things we should not, even as the body "wills" what it should not. In light of Jesus's humanity, Barth calls this disorder the sin of sloth (*Trägheit*).[29] In sloth we refuse our own humanity as it confronts us in Jesus Christ, a refusal that affects our relationships with God, ourselves, and others, including the relationship between our body and our soul.

One of the main characteristics of this body / soul disorder, says Barth, is dissatisfaction with our current life span. As it relates to the body and soul, sloth takes the unique form of "care" or "anxiety" with respect to our limited life span. In our sloth, says Barth, "we fret at the inevitable realization that our existence is limited. We would rather things were different. We try to arrest the foot which brings us constantly nearer to this frontier."[30] Moreover, in this state of dissipation and disintegration, we cannot understand that our desires cannot be satisfied. Barth says that "there is no infinite to satisfy our infinite desires. But this is something which the dissipated man, who has broken loose from the unity and totality of soul and body in which God has created him for existence in the limit of his time, cannot grasp, but must endlessly repudiate in his own endless dissatisfaction. In what he takes to be his successful hunt, he is himself the one who is hunted with terrible success by anxiety."[31] Thus Barth sees our concern over our limited existence as stemming from a fundamental disorder or disintegration between our body and soul, understood as the sin of sloth, an estimation made in light of

Jesus's real humanity. It should also be pointed out that sloth is not laziness; in fact it may often, says Barth, "disguise itself as ceaseless activity."[32]

Indeed, Barth might suggest that the separation of body and soul is very evident in the current attempts to extend the human life span and put off death indefinitely. Viewed in light of Athanasius's anthropology, current attempts to produce a pill that mimics the longevity effects of fasting without the downside of having to eat less or engage in fasting suggest that the body and the soul remain disintegrated and disordered, as the moral force of the body itself is dissolved, divided into a myriad of genetic pathways that will one day succumb to our technological control. The sentiment that a restriction in one's food intake will adversely affect the quality of one's life reveals that the body has little role to play in the development of one's character, and merely underscores that the body and soul have already gone their separate ways. More broadly, a Christian critique of the transhumanist goal of indefinite or even moderate life extension must ask what significance, if any, the body has for the transformation of one's soul or character in light of God in the flesh, the real man Jesus, who remains seated at the right hand of God.

If Athanasius's reflections on the first Adam remind us *positively* that the process of slowing aging is inextricably intertwined with the moral project of bringing one's body under the control of one's Word-guided soul, Barth's reflections on the second Adam, the real man Jesus, whose perfectly ordered soul and body lead to a life of obedience to God marked by death on the cross, remind us *negatively* that modifying the body to allay fears of death and aging can never effectively mitigate the fear that dwells in one's soul. It further suggests that Christians who choose to engage in regular fasting and thereby increase their chances for an extended life, might, somewhat paradoxically, become the kinds of people for whom an extended life is no longer a driving (much less ultimate) concern.

Conclusion

The transhumanist vision is built on the premise that death is the greatest enemy, an affront to human existence as we know it, and thus an enemy that must be defeated by knowledge. The Christian faith, too, sees death as an enemy. However, death in the Christian tradition is inextricably intertwined with both knowledge and sin. Indeed, it is good to be reminded that the tree of knowledge is also known as the "tree of disobedience."[33] Two centuries after Athanasius, Maximus the Confessor asserted that the fruit of this tree was a *theosis* of sorts, "a divinization of the creature, a self-love, a self-worship."[34] In light of the Christian narrative as expounded by Athanasius and

Barth, which is bounded by a garden at one end and the future resurrection at the other—a future opened up to us through the resurrection and ascension of Jesus Christ—could it be that transhumanism has confused the tree of knowledge with the tree of life, from which we have been cut off, but which came later in the form of the cross, through which death has already been conquered? To assert as much is not to deny the quest for a longer, healthier life, but it is to subsume this quest under the greater goal of being formed in Christ's image through embodied practices that recognize that the Incarnation bespeaks the goodness of embodiment, as we work toward that future where we will behold God in his glory—not as disembodied souls or uploaded minds—but as living, embodied beings who will continue to image the One who eternally bears the bodily scars that lead to eternal life.

Notes

1. See www.demog.berkeley.edu/~andrew/1918/figure2.html; and www .cia.gov/cia/publications/factbook/geos/us.html, as quoted by Fukuyama, *Our Posthuman Future*, 57. In the United States the life expectancy for babies born in 2000 was 79.6 and 73.5 years for females and males, respectively. At the Humanity+ Summit at Harvard University on June 13, 2010, the transhumanist Hank Hyena referred to Jeanne Calment as the "poster girl for longevity" and praised the "French way" in which she lived so long: "No caloric restriction. No supplement ingestion. Madame Jeanne ate 2 pounds of chocolate a week and she smoked cigarettes daily. . . . She never worked a day in her life—we hear that people should not retire, because they'll get bored and die, but Jeanne had a life of leisure day after day after day after day after day" (http://sites.google.com/site/hedonistfuturist/home/global-transhumanist-report).

2. Nagle, *View from Nowhere*, 224.

3. Aeschylus, *Prometheus Bound*, 248–53.

4. Robert Sokolowski writes that "this combination of assurance and blindness is necessary to men as a spur to use fire, and all that fire allows, to hold off death as long as possible." Sokolowski, *God of Faith and Reason*, 14.

5. Bartke et al., "Extending the Lifespan of Long-Lived Mice," 412.

6. Partridge and Gems, "Mechanisms of Ageing." The life span was increased from thirty-one days to just under two hundred days.

7. Guarente and Kenyon, "Genetic Pathways," 261.

8. This statement was made by S. Jay Olshansky during a presentation to the President's Council on Bioethics, "Session 2: Duration of Life: Is There a Biological Warranty Period?" December 12, 2002, www.bioethics.gov/transcripts/march03/session2.html. Olshansky asserts that "aging should be the enemy, not death. Going after the aging process itself, I think is fundamental."

9. Several have noted the current battles for legitimacy and "orthodoxy" within the field of gerontology. See Juengst et al., "Biogerontology."

10. See Kurzweil, "Human Body Version 2.0"; and Kurzweil, *Age of Spiritual*

Machines. Cf. Moravec, *Mind Children*; and Moravec, *Robot.* Also see de Grey, *Strategies for Engineered Negligible Senescence.*

11. Daniel Callahan noted that the Alliance for Aging Research reported the existence of twenty-five firms devoted to aging research, or "gero-techs," in 2000. See Perry, "Rise of the Gero-Techs."

12. Young, *Designer Evolution*, 40.

13. Ibid., 41.

14. Ibid., 43, 395.

15. Bacon, *History of Life and Death*, 467, states: "For, though we Christians do continually aspire and pant after the land of promise, yet it will be a token of God's favour towards us in our journeyings through this world's wilderness, to have our shoes and garments (I mean those of our frail bodies) little worn or impaired." See also the very insightful study by McKenny, *To Relieve the Human Condition.* McKenny describes the modern biomedical project or "Baconian Project" as the elimination of suffering and the expansion of choice.

16. Bacon, *Valerius Terminus*, 188–89. See also Rossi, *Francis Bacon*, 127.

17. Kärkkäinen, *One with God*, traces the development and expression of *theosis* from the early church fathers to contemporary Pentecostalism, focusing in particular on the Finnish School's interpretation of Luther's theology, as expounded by Tuomo Mannermaa. See Braaten and Jenson, *Union with Christ.* Although Aquinas never invoked the term *theosis*, he does describe the Christian life in terms of "participation" (2 Pt 1:4) in his discussion of the theological virtues, most significantly in the *Summa Theologica*, IaIIae, q. 62–63. See also Cavanaugh, "A Joint Declaration?"

18. Athanasius, *On the Incarnation*, 20, 38; Athanasius, *Four Discourses against the Arians*, 1.4, 1.60, 2.69, 3.3; and Athanasius, *Defence of the Nicene Definition*, 14. Norman Russell has helpfully observed that Athanasius develops two understandings of deification—ontological and ethical *theosis*—in parallel. Thus, Athanasius speaks of ontological deification as involving the objective work of Christ in divinizing human flesh by having assumed a human body—something however only to be fully realize at the resurrection—and he also speaks of ethical deification occurring through the ascetic and contemplative life. Hence, "the eschatological nature of deification does not mean that its beginnings are not discernable in this life." Russell, *Doctrine of Deification*, 9, 184.

19. Athanasius, *Incarnation*, 54.3, p. 65.

20. Burton-Christie, *Word in the Desert*, 222. The heading of the section from which this quotation was taken is titled "Freedom from Care."

21. O'Donovan, "Keeping Body and Soul Together," 232; emphasis added.

22. Barth, *Church Dogmatics*, vol. III, part 2 (hereafter *CD* III/2), 46.

23. Torrance, *Trinitarian Faith*, 150.

24. Price, *Karl Barth's Anthropology*, 9, 20–22, and esp. 234–44. However, Price notes that the term "dynamic anthropology" primarily applies to Barth's understanding of the *imago Dei* in view of the relational aspect of the Trinity (pp. 9–10). McLean, *Humanity in the Thought of Karl Barth*, 13; i.e., "No part [body or soul]

can be understood without the other, although distinctions are made and priorities given. There is unity, difference and order," 44.

25. Barth, *CD* III/2, 327. Barth derives this from Gal 1:4 and 2:20, where Jesus gave himself for our sins, giving up his soul for us (Mt 20:28; Jn 10: 11, 15; 1 Jn 3:16) and his body for us (Lk 22:19; Heb 10:10), *CD* III/2, 328ff.

26. Barth, *CD* III/2, 338; see also 336.

27. Ibid., 338.

28. Ibid., 339.

29. Sloth affects our relationship with God and is manifest as "stupidity"; our relationship with others, manifest as "inhumanity"; our relationship with ourselves, manifest as "dissipation"; and finally our relationship with time, manifest as "care" or "anxiety."

30. Barth, *Church Dogmatics*, vol. IV, part 2, 468.

31. Ibid., 463.

32. Ibid., 439.

33. Maximus the Confessor, *Quaestiones ad Thalasium*, prologue 260A.

34. Sherwood, "Introduction," 65, referring to Maximus, *Quaestiones ad Thalasium*, prologue 260A.

References

Aeschylus. *Prometheus Bound*, translated and edited by A. J. Podlecki. Oxford: Oxbow Books, 2005.

Aquinas, Thomas. *Summa Theologica*, translated by Fathers of the English Dominican Province. 5 vols. New York: Benziger Brothers, 1948.

Athanasius. *Defence of the Nicene Definition*. In *Nicene and Post-Nicene Fathers*, 2nd series, vol. 4, *Select Works and Letters*, edited by Philip Schaff and Henry Wace. New York: Christian Literature Co., 1892.

———. *Four Discourses against the Arians*. In *Nicene and Post-Nicene Fathers*, 2nd series, vol. 4, *Select Works and Letters*, edited by Philip Schaff and Henry Wace. New York: Christian Literature Co., 1892.

———. *Incarnation of the Word*. In *Nicene and Post-Nicene Fathers*, 2nd series, vol. 4, *Select Works and Letters*, edited by Philip Schaff and Henry Wace. New York: Christian Literature Co., 1892.

———. *Life of Antony*. In *Nicene and Post-Nicene Fathers*, 2nd series, vol. 4, *Select Works and Letters*, edited by Philip Schaff and Henry Wace. New York: Christian Literature Co., 1892.

Bacon, Francis. *History of Life and Death: The Prolongation of Human Life*. In *The Works of Francis Bacon, Lord Chancellor of England*, vol. 3, translated by Basil Montagu. Philadelphia: M. Murphy, 1876.

———. *Valerius Terminus*. In *The Philosophical Works of Francis Bacon, Baron of Verulam, Viscount St. Alban, and Lord High Chancellor of England*, edited by John M. Robertson, James Spedding, and Robert Leslie Ellis. London: George Routledge and Sons, 1905.

Barth, Karl. *Church Dogmatics*, edited by G. W. Bromiley and T. F. Torrance. 14 vols. Edinburgh: T. & T. Clark, 1936–69.

Bartke, Andre, Christ Wright, Julie A. Mattison, Donald K. Ingram, Richard A. Miller, and George S. Roth. "Extending the Lifespan of Long-Lived Mice." *Nature* 414 (2001): 412.

Braaten, Carl E., and Robert W. Jenson, eds. *Union with Christ: The New Finnish Interpretation of Luther*. Grand Rapids: William B. Eerdmans, 1998.

Burton-Christie, Douglas. *The Word in the Desert: Scripture and the Quest for Holiness*. Oxford: Oxford University Press, 1993.

Cavanaugh, William T. "A Joint Declaration?: Justification as Theosis in Aquinas and Luther." *Heythrop Journal* 41 (2000): 265–80.

de Grey, Aubrey S., ed. *Strategies for Engineered Negligible Senescence: Why Genuine Control of Aging May Be Foreseeable*. New York: New York Academy of Sciences, 2004.

Fukuyama, Francis. *Our Posthuman Future: Consequences of the Biotechnology Revolution*. New York: Farrar, Straus & Giroux, 2002.

Guarente, Leonard, and Cynthia Kenyon. "Genetic Pathways that Regulate Ageing in Model Organisms." *Nature* 408 (2000): 261.

Humanity+. "Transhumanist Declaration," 1998, 2009. http://humanityplus.org/learn/philosophy/transhumanist-declaration.

Juengst, Eric T., Robert H. Binstock, Maxwell Mehlman, Stephen G. Post, and Peter Whitehouse. "Biogerontology, 'Anti-Aging Medicine,' and the Challenges of Human Enhancement." *Hasting Center Report* 33 (2003): 21–30.

Kärkkäinen, Veli-Matti. *One with God: Salvation as Deification and Justification*. Collegeville, MN: Liturgical Press, 2004.

Klein, Bruce J., ed. *The Scientific Conquest of Death: Essays on Infinite Lifespans*. Buenos Aires: Libros EnRed, 2004.

Kurzweil, Ray. *The Age of Spiritual Machines: When Computers Exceed Human Intelligence*. New York: Penguin Books, 2000

———. "Human Body Version 2.0." in *The Scientific Conquest of Death: Essays on Infinite Lifespans*, edited by Bruce J. Klein. Buenos Aires: Libros EnRed, 2004.

Maximus the Confessor. *Quaestiones ad Thalasium*, edited by Carl Laga and Carlos Steel. Turnhout, Belgium: Brepols Publishers, 1980.

McKenny, Gerald P. *To Relieve the Human Condition: Bioethics, Technology, and the Body*. Albany: State University of New York Press, 1997.

McLean, Stuart. *Humanity in the Thought of Karl Barth*. Edinburgh: T. & T. Clark, 1981.

Moravec, Hans. *Mind Children: The Future of Robotic and Human Intelligence*. Cambridge, MA: Harvard University Press, 1988.

———. *Robot: Mere Machines to Transcendent Mind*. Oxford: Oxford University Press, 1999.

Nagle, Thomas. *The View from Nowhere*. Oxford: Oxford University Press, 1986.

O'Donovan, Oliver. "Keeping Body and Soul Together." In *On Moral Medicine: Theological Perspectives in Medical Ethics*, edited by Steven E. Lammers and Allen Verhey. Grand Rapids: William B. Eerdmans, 1998.

Partridge, L., and D. Gems. "Mechanisms of Ageing: Public or Private?" *Nature Reviews Genetics* 3 (2002): 165–75.

Perry, Daniel. "The Rise of the Gero-Techs." *Genetic Engineering News* 20 (2000): 57–58.

Price, Daniel J. *Karl Barth's Anthropology in Light of Modern Thought*. Grand Rapids: William B. Eerdmans, 2002.

Rossi, Paolo. *Francis Bacon: From Science to Magic*, translated by Sacha Rabinovich. London: Routledge & Kegan Paul, 1968.

Russell, Norman. *The Doctrine of Deification in the Greek Patristic Tradition*. Oxford: Oxford University Press, 2004.

Sherwood, Polycarp. "Introduction." In *St. Maximus the Confessor*, edited by Polycarp Sherwood. Westminster, MD: Newman Press, 1955.

Sokolowski, Robert. *The God of Faith and Reason: Foundations of Christian Theology*, 2nd ed. Washington, DC: Catholic University of America Press, 1995.

Torrance, Thomas F. *The Trinitarian Faith*. Edinburgh: T. & T. Clark, 1988.

Young, Simon. *Designer Evolution: A Transhumanist Manifesto*. Amherst, NY: Prometheus Books, 2006.

Chapter Ten

Human or Vulcan?

Theological Consideration of Emotional Control Enhancement

MICHAEL L. SPEZIO

Failures, things going wrong, can't shake the world's confidence in the necessity of its course and its development; such things are accepted with fortitude and sobriety as part of the bargain.
> —Dietrich Bonhoeffer, *Letters and Papers from Prison*, 3/161, 426

Be all that you can be—and a lot more.
> —Motto, Defense Sciences Office, US Defense
> Advanced Research Projects Administration

Transhumanism encompasses a wide variety of views generally oriented toward "the possibility and desirability of fundamentally improving the human condition through applied reason, especially by developing and making widely available technologies to eliminate aging and greatly enhance human intellectual, physical, and psychological capacities."[1] So claims Nick Bostrom, the executive director of the World Transhumanist Association, now known as Humanity+ (www.humanityplus.org). Bostrom, a professor of applied ethics at Oxford and the director of Oxford's Future of Humanity Institute, is one of the original cofounders of the World Transhumanist Association and is currently on its board of directors as founding chair. Depending upon which understanding of "human" one endorses, transhumanist visions either involve a stark contradiction in terms (for how can one *improve* the *human* condition by a project that seeks to bring about a *posthuman* future?) or the only logical result of a coherent if limited view of what is meant by "human." Ray Kurzweil, for example, believes that there is no contradiction in terms because humans are defined by "our ability to reach beyond our limitations," and so becoming posthuman is a very human thing to do. In this respect, Kurzweil's view is widely shared by transhumanists.

Though often overlooked, a significant transhumanist goal involves enhancing psychological capacities and "mental energy."[2] Often, such advocacy of psychological enhancement by transhumanists explicitly means complete or partial control of one's emotional life. Sometimes this means eliminating or controlling negative emotions, and sometimes it refers to the full, willful regulation of emotions of all kinds. So-called negative emotions, such as guilt, sadness, fear, and grief, are seen as unwanted, with no beneficial role. These negative emotions are often the focus of transhumanist projects and are slated for either elimination or full control in order to achieve the complete elimination of all suffering. Though most transhumanists no longer claim that all suffering can be eliminated, they are sure that negative emotions have no good role to play in a posthuman future.

These positions about the largely maladaptive role of emotion in relation to the human condition can be called "eliminationist" if they want to eliminate most or all emotional life, or "hemiemotionalist" if they want to only suppress or control the negative emotions. Both types are familiar to viewers of the original television series *Star Trek*, with its portrayal of the character of Spock, the first officer of the starship *Enterprise*. Spock is a "Vulcan," a humanoid species from a distant planet. As the story goes, the Vulcans barely survived a period of destruction due to their failure to control intense negative emotions, particularly grief and anger. To preserve their civilization, the Vulcans learned to suppress their emotions almost completely so that all situations and relations could be seen in the light of cold reason alone. Spock, however, is the son of a human mother and Vulcan father, a transhuman who successfully learned to be a Vulcan. His struggle to maintain a truly Vulcan emotional life, which is a challenge because of his human heritage via his very human mother, is a theme throughout the series and the later films. "Vulcanized" humans, then, would be those whose emotions have been significantly or completely eliminated. The series' association of emotion with weakness of will and a lack of rationality, and the association of such "weakness" with women and motherhood, is reflective of perspectives that, sadly, still shape current discourse about emotion in human life. One might think that such antifeminist, antiwomanist, and antiemotionalist biases would be rejected out of hand.

This is not true, however, and so this chapter seeks to engage, both theologically and scientifically, the strongly eliminationist and/or hemiemotionalist transhumanist project of emotional control enhancement currently being advanced by the Defense Advanced Research Projects Administration (DARPA). DARPA has made many public statements about the need to eliminate or strictly control negative emotions during war as it pursues its mission to develop what has been termed a "guilt-free soldier."[3] The case I argue against DARPA's eliminationist agenda is simple: Emotion makes us strong, not weak. Eliminating emotion will make us less human, not more human or rational, and certainly not transhuman in any sense of that word that is close to what the strongest advocates of transhumanism envision. I base this argument on a theological perspective best articulated by the German theologian Dietrich Bonhoeffer. My argument actually allies itself with certain central aspects of mainstream transhumanist projects, particularly in recognizing and emphasizing human strengths instead of weaknesses. DARPA's vision of the trans/posthuman "war fighter," I show, actually runs counter to the most prevalent transhumanist aspirations with regard to enhancing the human condition. After detailing aspects of DARPA's emotional control agenda, I argue for a theological response to such vulcanization that is as committed to humanity's strengths, to its mature condition (*mündigkeit*), as is transhumanism. However, the theological view I detail is more realistic than transhumanism about the centrality of relationality to human and posthuman goods and more inclined toward serious engagement of scientific accounts of human relationality, such as those of evolutionary biology, and social and affective neuroscience.

DARPA's Mission to "Weaken the Memory of Horrendous Acts"

DARPA's mission to "weaken the memory of horrendous acts,"[4] by engineering the remorseless war fighter, a person beyond the reach of posttraumatic stress disorder and the memories that are its cause, began primarily under the leadership of Tony Tether, DARPA's longest-running director in fifty years, who headed the agency from 2001 to 2009.[5] In 2002, soon after taking DARPA's helm, Tether memorably stated the goal for the enhanced human war fighter: "Imagine a warrior with the intellect of a human and the immortality of a machine."[6] Currently, one of DARPA's main projects along these lines is the REPAIR (Reorganization and Plasticity to Accelerate Injury Recovery) project, whose aim is to allow computer chips embedded in the human brain to directly alter directly the information processing in neural tissue.[7] According to the Stanford University researcher Krishna Shenoy, a professor of electrical and bioengineering who is funded by REPAIR, the goal is "to understand—and then be able to change—how the brain responds to trauma" via computational commands directly to brain tissue itself.[8] These commands are not first and foremost instructions to repair tissue. Rather, their aim is to change a person's memories, thoughts, and especially emotions via direct neural control. Though the therapeutic aims of this project are admirable, the technologies involved have broad implications for reducing or eliminating altogether such negative emotions as remorse or guilt over killing innocent civilians, anger at injustices, and regret about the mistreatment or abuse of prisoners.

Researchers sometimes recognize the potential ethical problems raised by DARPA's human enhancement mission, though often the ethical issues are minimized due to a misunderstanding of the ethical concerns themselves. For example, James McGaugh, a professor of neuroscience at the University of California, Irvine, and a leading scholar of emotional memory, denies that there is any moral quandary raised by eliminating memories or emotions. He likens the computational or pharmaceutical control of memories and emotions to giving penicillin in the case of a wound to the leg.[9] Conversely, Gregory Quirk, a professor of neuroscience at the University of Puerto Rico whose work has focused on how the brain overcomes fear conditioning, sees a potential for the misuse of emotion-control technologies. The use of such technologies to eliminate the emotions needed for morality, Quirk feels, would be objectionable.[10] Martha Farah, a professor of neuroscience at the University of Pennsylvania who has written on issues of neural enhancement and ethics, calls scientists to deeper engagement of these issues.[11] Meanwhile, a 2003 *Nature* editorial titled "Silence of the Neuroengineers" takes researchers to task for too willingly accepting DARPA funds without questioning the ultimate goals the agency has in mind. Stating bluntly that "researchers funded by a defense agency should stop skirting the ethical issues involved," the editorial criticizes scientists for generally "taking DARPA's money and citing possible medical benefits."[12]

Engaging Transhumanism as a Liberationist Movement

A promising approach to engaging transhumanist visions of this kind is to aim first at dialogue from a perspective that affirms human strength and potential as strongly as do the transhumanists themselves. For people of religious conviction to come to a better understanding of the transhumanist vision and to become more effective in shaping public policy, especially regarding brain-machine interfaces, I argue elsewhere for the need to engage the advocates of transhumanism in dialogue. I believe that a theological anthropology that emphasizes relationality and takes account of recent work in social neuroscience that supports the best of the transhuman vision will oppose such goals as the elimination of emotion.[13] Such an anthropology also figures largely in my argument here.

I begin by considering that transhumanist advocates see themselves as extensions of an Enlightenment project that advocates humanity's maturation and empowerment (*mündigkeit*) in throwing off a self-inflicted childishness or immaturity.[14] Such was Immanuel Kant's claim in his famous essay on the nature of enlightenment.[15] The organization Humanity+ sees the "Age of Enlightenment" as a critical stage in the history of transhumanist projects, as opposed to what they label as "bioconservatism," and the Marquis de Condorcet, arguably one of the earliest proponents of Enlightenment views, is quoted with approval on the Humanity+ website: "Nature has set no term to the perfection of human faculties."[16] Even transhumanism's most ardent critics acknowledge that it views itself as a liberation movement, standing in continuity with a tradition that has defended core human values.[17]

Kant wanted humans to stand on their own when thinking, to speak in their own voices when voicing public opinions, and to give up the *gängelwagen* (training-wheeled walkers) that hobble their thought. Transhumanists see humans with the condition known as "locked-in syndrome" being set free once again to speak via brain–machine interfaces. People who suffer from paralysis escape their wheelchairs in order to stand on their own, and all of us eventually leave behind the biological body due to what the transhumanists see as our many limiting disabilities, even when in perfect "health."[18] Kant thought that the process of moving from immaturity to *mündigkeit* is not easy, that it requires hard work and courage, and that at heart it is the formative process of making effective use of one's own understanding in addressing and responding to the public exchange of ideas.

Similarly, the transhumanists point to visions that require a courageous letting go of a biologically embodied humanity and a free striding into a new stage of human evolution, in which "the distinction between us and robots is going to disappear."[19] Granted, it is one thing to say that one may view transhumanism as descended from Enlightenment aspirations for human self-expression, and quite another to argue conclusively that this is the case. Here I attempt no such argument regarding the intellectual sources of transhumanism. The argument offered regarding the enhancement of emotional control, however, depends on granting transhumanism such standing as a rightful heir of the Enlightenment. Thus I take quite seriously the transhumanists' claims regarding their commitment to reasoned conversation and engagement in directing future applications of technology.[20]

Because of the strong similarities between Enlightenment notions of *mündigkeit* and transhumanist notions of living out the full extent of human potentiality, it really is unproductive to characterize transhumanist/posthumanist visions as somehow irrelevant because they are ultimately unrealistic, or as drawn from comic-book visions of human enhancement, or as impossible because of human limitation that will result in eventual failure. Indeed, as Bonhoeffer noted in his later theological anthropology, "fortitude and sobriety" at the prospect of failure is characteristic of mature humanity. How can such a humanity view those quick to paint nightmare scenarios of posthuman blight with anything but the deepest skepticism, and perhaps even pity? It is thus unhelpful for future decision making, in medicine or policy, to label transhumanism one of the world's most dangerous ideas—as Francis Fukuyama did—or to invoke demonic imagery immediately upon any consideration of neurocognitive enhancement beyond the neurotypical.[21] This approach is suggested in the comment of Leon Kass when he was the chair of the President's Council on Bioethics: "There's the question of desire and attention, and if we're going to do a kind of analysis of all of these things and find out, well, there's this piece which could enhance you slightly and you can take me to the next one, and before you know it I've given away the entire activity and we've got some kind of—the equivalent of some kind of little demon who's inside of me doing this."[22]

Such caricatures of core transhumanist projects might very well come to be seen as similar to what Byron L. Sherwin calls the "third phase" of the golem legend, which always depicts the nonhuman, artificial creation as dangerous, and which developed in the late nineteenth and early twentieth centuries, perhaps in response to increasing industrialization.[23] The two earlier phases, according to Sherwin, simply viewed the creation of golem as either an outflow of the *imago Dei*, in which humans are like God in their creative power, or as a response to a practical need, such as the protection of the innocent.[24] Interestingly, these earlier phases have obvious parallels in transhumanist claims.

Instead of painting doomsday scenarios, one might attempt postmodernist opposition to transhumanist projects, given transhumanism's self-described rootedness in and fulfillment of the grand metanarrative of Enlightenment thinking. Yet such approaches, though interesting, would ultimately fail due to the fact that transhumanism itself puts in serious question perhaps the grandest metanarrative of all, namely, the centrality of the known biological body to humanity and to personhood in general. Indeed, transhumanism could be characterized as learning from the genealogical investigations of Michel Foucault, specifically with respect to the questions about and consequences of defining human nature in any substantial way. Foucault strongly resisted naturalizing the question of the human, famously so in a debate with the linguist Noam Chomsky, and focused instead on the history of our concept of the human and what each new version entails for enacting power in and over human society.[25] Though transhumanists, to my knowledge, have not cast themselves as Foucaultian or as rooted in a genealogical approach to human nature, such a position is reasonable. Therefore, standard postmodern attacks on transhumanist projects will have difficulty succeeding.

In the end, to argue effectively against vulcanized or hemiemotionalized agendas of the posthuman, it is thus best to acknowledge the liberationist aspirations of transhumanism, as well as its descent from a tradition that has long sought the freedom of humanity from all forms of immaturity and intellectual slavery. Transhumanism, seen as a liberationist movement born out of Enlightenment commitments to clear and unbiased intellectual exploration, seeks to view humanity "as we truly are," so as to fully actualize human potential through technology.[26]

However, central to any complete concept of humanity is relationality. Any view of the human that marginalizes or denigrates relationality risks being itself marginalized as pure fiction or as denying that which belongs to the core of human strength and maturity. Further, relationality entails the friendship, love, empathy, compassion, nurture, and care that transhumanists see as the individual and social goods so strongly justifying the posthuman future.[27] Yet such goods, and even rationality itself, depend upon a full and rich emotional life, as shown by recent work in the neuroscience of decision making. What is needed, then, is a theological vision that affirms relationality even as it stands completely with transhumanism in the celebration of human maturation and strength. Such a theology is found in the later writings of Dietrich Bonhoeffer.

Mündigkeit and Relationality in the Theology of Dietrich Bonhoeffer

Bonhoeffer, who is perhaps best remembered for his perceived close association with Karl Barth and Protestant neoorthodoxy early in his theological career, and for his imprisonment and death by the Nazi regime in Germany, may seem an odd theological partner for a dialogue with transhumanism. Yet he was a clear witness to human freedom of conscience, grounded in faith in God. From his cell in Tegel Prison, he questioned whether humans without knowledge of the "sphere of freedom" or "play space" could really be "full human being[s]" or even "Christian in the fullest sense."[28] The church was to be the new place of freedom's founding, quite in contrast to its primary association with obedience. Perhaps as a consequence of his sense of freedom in faith, which was already evident in his doctoral dissertation and habilitation, in the end he wholly rejected Barth's "positivism of revelation," saying that "nothing decisive has been gained here," and even going so far as to call Barth's overreliance on revelation "not biblical."[29] He wanted no part of a dogmatic statement that Christian teaching is beyond the world's investigation and stands apart from worldviews characteristic of mature human thought.

Beyond the witness of Bonhoeffer's life, his written theology emphasizing a mature turn toward committed fellowship in discipleship, and his clear break with Barth, three key aspects more prominently emphasized in his later theology—which are sometimes characterized as a "new humanism"—make it an apt partner in dialogue with transhumanism.[30] First, he wholly embraced mature humanity and continually spoke of Christian theology needing to take account of a world "come of age." Second, he was completely open to scientific research and its implications for human understanding of both human and nonhuman nature. This was likely due to his close relationship with his brother, Karl Friedrich, a secular humanist who was appointed the director of the Max-Planck Institute for Physical Chemistry in Göttingen after the war. It was his brother who recommended that he read Carl Friedrich von Weizsäcker's *Worldview of Physics*, which convinced him even more of the world's *mündigkeit* and solidified his view that God can never be viewed as filling epistemological gaps.[31] Third and finally, as one who took seriously the need to see humans as they are, he made relationality central to his theology and his theological anthropology. The first two aspects serve to establish his rapport with transhumanist perspectives on the human condition, and the third provides useful and reasoned opposition to transhumanist views that have an unrealistic or anemic view of the human and of the complexity of human society.

Bonhoeffer's later theological anthropology and ecclesiology strongly condemned any attempt by Christianity or other religions to prey upon humanity's finitude and supposed weaknesses as an apologetic strategy for establishing a *need* for God. Amazingly, his attitude toward scholars or clergy who attempt "to prove to secure, contented, and happy human beings that they are in reality miserable and desperate" was harsh: "Where there is health, strength, security, and simplicity, these experts scent sweet fruit on which they can gnaw or lay their corrupting eggs. They set about to drive people to inner despair, and then they have a game they can win."[32]

These remarks appeared in the same letter (to Eberhard Bethge, June 8, 1944) in which Bonhoeffer first used the term *mündigkeit* and first spoke of the world's coming of age in this way. In a letter only a few weeks later, he spoke approvingly of theology that constructs divinity "from the riches and depth of existence rather than from its cares and longings."[33] In light of his anthropology, he characterized the false focus on human weakness as "first of all, pointless, second, ignoble, and third, unchristian." They were pointless because the so-called weaknesses no longer existed; ignoble because they hit people when they were down, committing "so to speak, religious rape"; and unchristian because they identified the power of Christ with a withdrawal from the world rather than with enthusiastic membership in it. He called the identification of humanity with weakness and dependence upon God a distinctly "religious" viewpoint, and in rejecting it calls for a "religionless Christianity," understood as Christianity in the world as if God were not present in it.[34]

Instead of *human* weakness, in religionless Christianity it is *God* who is weak and suffering and who "gains ground and power in the world by being powerless."[35] God's ground and power, interpreted in this way, are the drawing together of those who identify as Christians and those who identify as awakened and mature in the world. No longer is there an inner spiritual space that Christians can keep pure, and that the church is called to keep holy. In the new religionless Christianity, the silence and suffering of God, God's weakness, draws Christians to the true suffering that exists in the world, and to those persons who really suffer, freeing Christians from continually wanting to expose putative weaknesses in others so as to find room for God.

This brief analysis has three implications for future theological engagement with transhumanism. First, it is clear that transhumanism's emphasis on the use of technology for alleviating human disability, pain, despair, and social isolation has a strong theological grounding and support. Bonhoeffer also pointed out that "never did Jesus question anyone's health and strength or good fortune as such or regard it as rotten fruit; otherwise why would he have made sick people well or given strength back to the weak?"[36] Second, as transhumanism aspires to alleviate the suffering and social disruption caused by human limitations that are not as yet widely viewed as human disabilities (e.g., the upper limit of the human lifespan at about 120 years), theology again can save Christians from too keen a hunger for human weakness and finitude. Christians can be freed from anxieties over trespassing against so-called divinely ordained limitations and given courage to explore when the limitations of human biology may be transcended through technology. Third, a theology coming from a religionless Christianity stands courageously, yet with some sure fellow-feeling, against transhumanist trends that ignore real and widespread suffering in order to go on building a rarified and restricted posthuman perfection.

Bonhoeffer's openness to science and scientific worldviews deserves a brief mention, if only because this is another way in which his later theology is both similar to mainstream transhumanism and wholly dissimilar to the Barthian neoorthodoxy with which he is so often identified. Bonhoeffer explicitly rejected any attempt to argue against scientific findings on the grounds that by so doing one might better defend God's place in the world. Instead, he wanted Christians to "find God in what we know, not in what we don't know; God wants to be grasped by us not in unsolved questions but in those that have been solved. This is true of the relation between God and scientific knowledge."[37] He voiced these reflections while reading *Worldview of Physics*, and he clearly saw, in the work and ethical dedication of his older brother, the physicist and agnostic Karl Friedrich, a compelling way of being a both a scientist and a courageous resister of oppression in the world. Of particular importance for Bonhoeffer, his engagement with physics and with his brother led to a theology whereby God must be seen as the "center of life." This meant for him and for his lifelong theology that God is the basis of relationality and is present in relationality.

Bonhoeffer's view of ethics as formation is one of the best ways of understanding how central a role relationality had within his theology and theological anthropology. For him, moral and ethical choice emerged not from aspects external to relationship, such as brute consequences or heteronomous duty, but as involving and requiring first and always a commitment of being-in-relationship. Though more than ten years separate the publication of his early work on the church, *Sanctorum Communio*, and his *Ethics*, Bonhoeffer kept in mind all along an account of human nature that focuses on identity formed in relation.[38] For him ethics and questions of value can only be understood in terms of identity-in-relationality, ultimately with the divine, but not separated from the community to which and for which one is responsible. For him personhood emerges only through encounters with the other, only when the "moment" involves certainty of knowledge about this or that characteristic of the other, and only when the moment forms a direct acknowledgment of the other, in which one is called to "believe in" the other.[39]

In this way Bonhoeffer rejects the notion that humans are persons only if they have the potential or actual capacity to participate in reason and thus in universals. Such capacitative ways of defining humanity continue to confront us today in ways that are significant for engaging transhumanism, from Martha Nussbaum's "capabilities" theory of flourishing to Peter Singer's fierce arguments against what he calls "speciesism" to Robert George's passionate argument in favor of reason suppressing all emotional impulses that would lead us ethically astray from our true duty. Bonhoeffer also rejects Epicureanism for its utilitarian foundations, in which the other is a means to an end and in which happiness or pleasure must be understood as divisible into each individual. This approach, he claims, critically disallows any consideration of a relational good, such that "there are no essential or meaningful relations between human beings that are grounded in the human spirit; connections to others are not intrinsic but only utilitarian."[40] He cites Hobbes's *Leviathan* here, via Kant's *Religion within the Limits of Reason Alone*, to suggest that under this system, all relational forms are purely contractual and satisfy self-interest, enlightened though such self-interest may be. Finally, he rejects what he sees as Descartes's error in focusing too much on epistemology, such that the standards of theoretical reason are substituted for a proper understanding of practical reason. Here, Bonhoeffer traces this error through Kant and Fichte, identifying it as substituting instrumental, procedural conceptions of reason, which may work well in the purely theoretical domain, for more metaphysically grounded conceptions of practical reason. Bonhoeffer's concern is to reject the utilitarian tendency of theoretical reasons in favor of a relational, practical reason, which enables recognition of the good and encourages a disposition for virtue.

Throughout these rejections, Bonhoeffer opposes any approach that makes the existence of, the responsibility for, and the encounter with the other purely incidental to morality, an effect or situation to be managed rather than a constitutive element within the moral attitude. Relying so heavily on theoretical reason in the moral domain reduces the other to an object and as at most a very important aspect in some formal moral calculus, but certainly something much less than a person in Bonhoeffer's conception.

This debate surrounding the place of a procedural, instrumental view of reason within theories of moral action (i.e., practical reason) continues today.[41] In this assessment of Bonhoeffer's contribution to the debate, it is important to recognize that from his initial work in *Communio* to his final conception in the *Ethics*, he rejects the conflation of theoretical and practical reason and denies that practical reason can or should be modeled on theoretical reason. He writes in the *Communio*: "It is impossible to reach the real existence of other subjects by way of the purely transcendental category of the universal. . . . As long as my intellect is dominant, exclusively claiming universal validity, as long as all contradictions that can arise when one knows a subject as an object of knowledge are conceived as immanent to my intellect, I am not in the social sphere."[42]

Not surprisingly, in his manuscript titled "Ethics as Formation," the first ethical failure Bonhoeffer identifies is the failure of reasonable people, or those seeking to be only guided by cold reason alone, to be ethical apart from any emotional tie. Bonhoeffer writes this while deeply involved, with his close friends and family, in the struggle to resist the Nazi regime. Those guided by reason alone, as he calls them, might also be seen as the "vulcanized" humans that we considered above. He accuses such "reasonable" people of ever striving but with "defective vision," and therefore either collapsing into apathy, "bitterly disappointed that the world is so unreasonable," or falling "helplessly captive to the stronger party."[43]

Bonhoeffer's emphasis on relationality and his close linkage of human relation to ethical formation are significant for our attempt at theological engagement with transhumanism. Perhaps most important, his theology, as much as it recognizes human autonomy and maturity, rejects an individualistic notion of these concepts. In this way, he resists the individualistic excesses of the Enlightenment, including any efforts to enhance reason by diminishing the emotional life that makes relationality possible. His approach allows a partnership with transhumanist projects that seek further human liberation, but his theology also helps refocus these projects on the critical nature of relationality to the transhuman/posthuman future. Thus, his theology reorients transhumanist projects toward a more realistic consideration of human strengths, including the possibility that emotional life, far from being a weakness, is one of humanity's greatest assets.

Relationality as Strength: The Social Brain and the Empathic Person

Given the discussion above, recent scientific research indeed seems consistent with Bonhoeffer's views and even with his central claims about relationality. First, evolutionary biology points to evidence that the human brain's evolution was strongly influenced by a need to develop relationality in the species. Second, neuroscience points to evidence that such relationality—including close bonding, friendship, nurture, and care—depends upon emotion. Relationality makes possible the adaptive trait of the rapid sharing of understanding that is critical to social ties. If anything, these scientific views affirm both the maturity and relationality of the human as found in Bonhoeffer's theology, suggesting that his account is closer to a realistic view of the human, and to transhumanist aspirations, than is the account motivating DARPA's vulcanization projects.

In evolutionary biology, the Social Brain Hypothesis states that humans and nonhuman primates in general have the kind of brains they have due to the need to function socially within community. That is, evolutionary pressures have resulted in larger brains and in information-processing networks so as to allow relatively rapid transformation of signals from the face, voice, posture, and movements into signals that convey goals, intentions, and emotions, or social understanding. Until recently, selective pressures were understood almost exclusively in terms of social competitiveness. Recent research, however, has demonstrated that the formation of close social bonds among two to five primates of the same species was at least as important, if not more so, for the selection of networks for social understanding.[44]

The ways in which shared understanding is supported by these networks involve what has become known as *simulation processes*. Simulation theories constructed from data demonstrating these processes make it clear that emotionally relevant conceptual processing is essential for adaptive and efficient social engagement.[45] Simulation theoretic frameworks in affective and social neuroscience identify similar processing involved in both the *experience* of an intention or emotion in oneself and the *perception* of an intention or emotion in another. The networks carrying out this double duty of self-representation and other-representation are termed "shared circuits" or sometimes "mirror neurons." These networks are then supportive of empathy, which is the ability to spontaneously and even subconsciously reconstruct in oneself what another is feeling, thinking, and intending.[46] Damage to the networks that contribute to the conceptualization of another's state of mind, intention, emotional outlook, and mood results in an inability to respond properly to others or to sense their joy or suffering. When occurring early in development, such damage can result in a violent psychopathy due to a complete absence of compassion. In other words, functioning emotions in oneself are required for an adequate understanding of those emotions in another.

The Transhuman Future: Relational, Emotional, and Empathic

It is now clear that Bonhoeffer's vision of relationality as central to humanity and his affirmation of human autonomy in relation is much closer to current scientific views of humanity than those views that see the possibility of a vulcanized transhuman future. Consider what would happen if transhumanist projects to vulcanize the posthuman succeeded. By allowing complete control over or elimination of negative emotions, it is very likely that these projects would severely limit a posthuman's ability to evaluate the suffering, pain, grief, sadness, fear, or anger of another person. Yet the stated goal of most transhumanist visions is to increase relationality and social understanding via enhanced empathy, compassion, nurture, and caring. Those so-called transhumanist programs that seek a vulcanization of the human have not paid close enough attention to human evolutionary biology or to the recent advances in affective and social neuroscience. They fail to engage the human sciences fully, and the result is an inability to see "ourselves as we really are." Further, vulcanized visions of the transhuman/posthuman ultimately undermine the main goals of liberation celebrated by transhumanism in the first place, which leads to the conclusion that vulcanization is not authentic transhumanism.

This can easily be seen by first noting that nearly every prevailing transhumanist program seeks to enhance the adaptive, efficient functioning of social systems. Indeed, such claims are growing ever stronger, as has been shown by recent justifications for transhumanist agendas. According to these justificatory arguments, without social enhancements in cross-cultural understanding, well-being, and peace seeking, the destruction of life due to nuclear war or climate catastrophe is assured. Yet, as Bonhoeffer argued and as contemporary science seems to support, there is no way to achieve social enhancement if transhumans or posthumans lack the ability to enter into relation and thus to perceive, rapidly and efficiently, the emotions in others, including and perhaps especially negative emotions. Even if it were possible to vulcanize or hemiemotionalize all persons at the same time, say through simultaneous somatic and germline alteration, the desired social enhancement would quickly disappear with any appearance of sadness, grief, fear, anger, pain, or suffering. Recall that the hope that a transhumanist/posthumanist future will result in a world free of suffering has long since been given up as completely unrealistic by all but the most extreme transhumanists.

Finally, consider again DARPA's desire for a better war fighter, one who would not suffer remorse or guilt or grief over any act of killing during war. Imagine the kinds of enhancements that would be required for a transhuman or posthuman not to feel any negative emotion in the wake of knowing either that one has killed innocent persons or that one has seen one's fellow soldier killed violently in front of one's eyes. Unemotional persons like this might indeed be spared the trauma of struggling with posttraumatic stress disorder, which is the stated goal. Yet the extremity of their "enhancements" would very likely render them unable to respond *relationally* and thus effectively to injuries sustained by fellow war fighters, not to mention their inability to deal adequately with civilian life.

Clearly, the theological perspective that I have drawn from Bonhoeffer is much more in line with transhumanism than is DARPA's vision of the enhanced war fighter. Furthermore, this theology demonstrates a much closer affinity to scientific thinking in evolutionary biology and in social and affective neuroscience than do vulcanizing visions of a posthuman future. Note also that the endorsement of relationality within the whole of Bonhoeffer's theology and his emphasis on human strengths and maturity corresponds to transhumanism. This correspondence is based on the fact that relationality is not viewed as human weakness by any coherent transhumanist program and that it is seen as a significant evolutionary advance within neuroscientific accounts of the human. Bonhoeffer's emphasis on God's suffering and on God's absence as presence provides a more realistic view of possible posthuman futures than is offered by the proponents of vulcanization. In his prison vision Bonhoeffer foresees how relationality and suffering—along with maturity, courage, and strength—are waiting for us in the world that lies in our future. Bonhoeffer's later theology encourages us to be free from concern over God's supposed exclusion from the world so that we may look for and respond to the suffering of others in the world, even while affirming those others as mature, autonomous, and strong children of God. Such theological engagement can only promote more effective future visions as we take up transhumanist dialogues.

Notes

The author acknowledges helpful comments by anonymous reviewers and support from the Science and Transcendence Advanced Research Series and the Center for Theology and the Natural Sciences.

1. Bostrom, "Transhumanism FAQ 2.1."

2. "Transhumanist Declaration," 2009, available at http://humanityplus.org.

3. Baard, "Guilt-Free Soldier."

4. Jim McGaugh, research professor of neurobiology and behavior at University of California, Irvine, and fellow of Irvine's Center for the Neurobiology of Learning and Memory, quoted by Baard, "Guilt-Free Soldier."

5. Shachtman, "Darpa Chief Speaks."

6. Harlow, "Meet the Cyborgs."

7. See www.darpa.mil/dso/solicitations/baa09-27.htm; and Drummond, "Pentagon Turns to Brain Implants."

8. Ibid.

9. Baard, "Guilt-Free Soldier."

10. Ibid.

11. See, e.g., Farah et al., "Neurocognitive Enhancement."

12. *Nature.* "Silence of the Neuroengineers,"

13. See Spezio, "Brain and Machine."

14. Bostrom, "Transhumanism FAQ 2.1."

15. Kant, "Answer to the Question."

16. Humanity+, http://humanityplus.org.au/about/. The comment from de Condorcet is found in his *Sketch for a Historical Picture of the Progress of the Human Mind,* 1795.

17. See Fukuyama, "World's Most Dangerous Ideas: Transhumanism."

18. Kurzweil, *Singularity,* 311.

19. Brooks, *Flesh and Machines.*

20. At times, however, transhumanist rhetoric undermines the stated goal of engaged dialogue. Transhumanist attempts to caricature opponents with such pejorative terms as "bioconservative," "vulgar prejudice," and "neoluddite" seriously detract from transhumanism's claimed aspirations of unbiased, enlightenment thinking.

21. Fukuyama, "World's Most Dangerous Ideas: Transhumanism."

22. Leon Kass, transcript, meeting of the President's Council on Bioethics, January 16, 2003, http://bioethics.georgetown.edu/pcbe/transcripts/jan03/session3.html.

23. See Sherwin, *Golems among Us,* 23, 45–46.

24. Ibid., 7–17, 45.

25. Chomsky and Foucault, *Chomsky–Foucault Debate.*

26. See Clark, *Natural-Born Cyborgs,* 198.

27. Bostrom and Sandberg, "Wisdom of Nature."

28. Bonhoeffer, *Letters and Papers,* 268.

29. Ibid., 364, 373.

30. Ibid., 28–30.

31. Ibid., 405–6. See also von Weizsäcker, *Worldview of Physics*, which Bonhoeffer described as a "philosophy of nature" (p. 104).

32. Bonhoeffer, *Letters and Papers*, 427.

33. Ibid., 440.

34. Ibid., 479.

35. Ibid., 480.

36. Ibid., 451.

37. Ibid., 406.

38. Bonhoeffer, *Sanctorum Communio*; Bonhoeffer, *Ethics*.

39. Bonhoeffer, *Sanctorum Communio*, 54.

40. Ibid., 39.

41. See Taylor, "Modern Moral Rationalism."

42. Bonhoeffer, *Sanctorum Communio*, 45.

43. Bonhoeffer, *Ethics*, 78.

44. Dunbar, "Social Brain"; Dunbar, "Social Role of Touch."

45. Adolphs, "How Do We Know the Minds of Others?"; Spezio, "Narrative in Holistic Healing"; Adolphs and Spezio, "Role of the Amygdala."

46. Singer and Lamm, "Social Neuroscience of Empathy."

References

Adolphs, R. "How Do We Know the Minds of Others? Domain-Specificity, Simulation, and Enactive Social Cognition." *Brain Research* 1079, no. 1 (2006): 25–35.

Adolphs, R., and M. Spezio. "Role of the Amygdala in Processing Visual Social Stimuli." *Progress in Brain Research* 156 (2006): 363–78.

Baard, Erik. "The Guilt-Free Soldier: New Science Raises the Specter of a World without Regret." *Village Voice*, January 21, 2003.

Bonhoeffer, Dietrich. *Ethics*, translated by Ilse Todt, Heinz Eduard Todt, Ernst Feil, and Clifford Green. Vol. 6 of *Dietrich Bonhoeffer's Works in English*. 16 vols. Minneapolis: Fortress, 2005 (orig. pub. 1949).

———. *Letters and Papers from Prison*, translated by Isabel Best, Lisa E. Dahill, Reinhard Krauss, Nancy Lukens, Martin Rumscheidt, and Barbara Rumscheidt; edited by Victoria J. Barnett and Barbara Wojhowski. Vol. 8 of *Dietrich Bonhoeffer's Works in English*. 16 vols. Minneapolis: Fortress Press, 2009.

———. *Sanctorum Communio: Theological Study of the Sociology of the Church*, translated by Reinhard Krauss and Nancy Lukens. Vol. 1 of *Dietrich Bonhoeffer's Works in English*. 16 vols. Minneapolis: Fortress, 1998.

Bostrom, Nick. "A History of Transhumanist Thought." *Journal of Evolution and Technology* 14, no. 1 (2005): 1.25.

———. "The Transhumanism FAQ 2.1." www.transhumanism.org.resources/ FAQv21.pdf

Bostrom, Nick, and Anders Sandberg. "The Wisdom of Nature: An Evolutionary Heuristic for Human Enhancement." In *Human Enhancement*, edited by

J. Savulescu and N. Bostrom. New York: Oxford University Press, 2008.

Brooks, Rodney. *Flesh and Machines: How Robots Will Change Us.* New York: Pantheon, 2002.

Chomsky, Noam, and Michel Foucault. *The Chomsky–Foucault Debate on Human Nature.* New York: New Press, 2006.

Clark, Andy. *Natural-Born Cyborgs: Minds, Technologies, and the Future of Human Intelligence.* New York: Oxford University Press, 2003.

Drummond, Katie. "Pentagon Turns to Brain Implants to Repair Damaged Minds." *Danger Room, Wired Magazine,* May 2010. www.wired.com/dangerroom/2010/05/pentagon-turns-to-brain-implants-to-repair-damaged-minds/#more-24419

Dunbar, R. I. M. "The Social Brain: Mind, Language, and Society in Evolutionary Perspective." *Annual Review of Anthropology* 32 (2003): 163–81.

———. "The Social Role of Touch in Humans and Primates: Behavioural Function and Neurobiological Mechanisms " *Neuroscience and Biobehavioral Reviews* 34, no. 2 (2008): 260–68.

Etzel, J. A., V. Gazzola, and C. Keysers. "Testing Simulation Theory with Cross-Modal Multivariate Classification of fMRI Data." *PLoS One* 3, no. 11 (2008): e3690.

Farah, Martha J., Judy Illes, Robert Cook-Degan, Howard Gardner, Eric Kandel, Patricia King, Erik Parens, Barbara Sahakian, and Paul Root Wolpe. "Neurocognitive Enhancement: What Can We Do and What Should We Do?" *Nature Reviews Neuroscience* 5 (2004): 421–25.

Fukuyama, Francis. "World's Most Dangerous Ideas: Transhumanism." *Foreign Policy* 144 (2004): 42–43.

Harlow, John. "Meet the Cyborgs: Humans with a Hint of Machine." *Sunday Times,* March 21, 2004.

Kant, Immanuel. "An Answer to the Question: What Is Enlightenment?" In *Practical Philosophy,* edited by Mary J. Gregor, 17–22. New York: Cambridge University Press, 1999.

Kurzweil, Ray. *The Singularity Is Near: When Humans Transcend Biology.* New York: Viking Press, 2005.

Nature. "Silence of the Neuroengineers." *Nature* 423 (2003): 787.

Shachtman, Noah. "Darpa Chief Speaks." *Danger Room, Wired Magazine,* February 2007. www.wired.com/dangerroom/2007/02/tony_tether_has_1/?intcid=postnav.

Sherwin, Byron L. *Golems among Us: How a Jewish Legend Can Help Us Navigate the Biotech Century.* Chicago: Ivan R. Dee, 2004.

Singer, T., and C. Lamm. "The Social Neuroscience of Empathy." *Annals of the New York Academy of Science* 1156 (2009): 81–96.

Spezio, Michael L. "Brain and Machine: Minding the Transhuman Future." *Dialog* 44 (2005): 375.

———. "Narrative in Holistic Healing: Empathy, Sympathy, & Simulation Theory." In *Spiritual Transformation and Healing,* edited by Joan D. Koss and Philip Hefner, 206–22. Lanham, MD: Altamira, 2006.

Taylor, Charles. "Modern Moral Rationalism." In *Weakening Philosophy: Essays in Honor of Gianni Vattimo*, edited by Santiago Zabala, 57–76. Montreal: McGill–Queen's University Press, 2007.

von Weizsäcker, Carl Friedrich. *The World View of Physics*. Trans. by Marjorie Grene. London: Routledge and K. Paul, 1952.

Chapter Eleven

Whose Salvation? Which Eschatology?

Transhumanism and Christianity as
Contending Salvific Religions

BRENT WATERS

For why should men fear to die, and prefer to live in . . . distress than
to end it by dying? The only reason is the obvious natural revulsion
from annihilation. And that is the reason why men, although they know
that they are destined to die, long for this mercy to be granted them,
as a great boon, the mercy, that is, of an extension of life in this pitiable
state, and the deferment of their death. This shows without any shadow
of doubt that they would grasp at the offer of immortality, with the
greatest delight, even an immortality which would offer no end to their
beggarly condition.

—Saint Augustine, *The City of God*, VI.27

The Greeks' concern with immortality grew out of their experience of
an immortal nature and immortal gods which together surrounded the
individual lives of mortal men. Imbedded in a cosmos where everything
was immortal, mortality became the hallmark of human existence. Men
are "the mortals," the only mortal things in existence, because unlike
animals they do not exist only as members of a species.

—Hannah Arendt, *The Human Condition*

Death, and more broadly finitude and mortality, has been a peren-
nial religious concern, a universal yet nonetheless anxiety-ridden
attribute of the human condition prompting some kind of salvific response.
These responses have ranged from indifferent resignation to desperate struggle. On the one hand, the Pre-Socratics share with Nietzsche an *amor fati*
that frees them from a hopeless struggle against a mortal fate that they cannot vanquish; on the other hand, the Aristotelians share with Hegel a hope
that this old enemy can be overcome through human work and history. It is
this latter response that concerns us in this chapter.

For the ancient Greeks, as Arendt indicates, the dilemma stemmed from
their perception of an immortal universe in which humans, as individuated

and self-aware beings, were the only mortal creatures. How could a mortal person somehow continue to participate in the world's endless time? The solution lay in contributing to works that transcended one's death, such as family and politics. A person could live on through an immortal lineage or empire—an effort refined, if not displaced, by the modern belief in an immortal history as the premier human work. In contrast, Christians believe that humans are part of a finite and temporal creation, but this does not relieve the anxiety of one's mortal fate. Death is the final enemy, and as Saint Augustine observed it is not unnatural that anyone would grasp at an offer of immortality or even a brief extension of life. For the Christian, finitude and mortality can only be overcome through death's penultimate victory, which is in turn reversed through one's resurrection into the eternal life of the triune God.

Transhumanism represents a late modern religious response to the finite and mortal constraints of human existence. It is not a religion in a formal sense, but as Martin Luther suggests, wherever one places one's confidence is necessarily one's god—or, more broadly, one's object of faith or ultimate concern.[1] In this respect, transhumanism and Christianity appear to have a number of similarities, particularly with regard to soteriology and eschatology. Transhumanists and Christians agree, for instance, that the finite and mortal human condition is far from ideal. For transhumanists humans have fallen short of achieving their true potential, whereas for Christians humans have not yet become the kinds of creatures God intends them to be. In response both agree that humans require release from their current condition. For transhumanists this release is attained through technological transformation, whereas for Christians humans are transformed by their life in Christ. Both agree that death is the final enemy; transhumanists conquer this foe by achieving the immortality of endless time, whereas Christians are resurrected into eternity, where there is no time. Consequently, both place their hope in a future that is speculative rather than concrete. Moreover, these similarities are apparently reinforced by selective Christian theological discourse, such as Pierre Teilhard de Chardin's vision of human evolution culminating in the Noosphere or Omega Point, and Philip Hefner's celebration of the cyborg.[2]

These similarities, however, are more apparent than substantive, for transhumanists draw their core beliefs and convictions often unwittingly from what Christians would regard as heretical sources. This observation regarding transhumanism's intellectual genealogy is not meant to be pejorative; identifying these sources for transhumanism does not automatically mean that its subsequent analysis of and proposed solution for relieving the human condition are necessarily wrong. Rather, it serves to demonstrate why Christian theology should greet transhumanism with at best skepticism and at worst grave caution. The purpose of this chapter is to explain why such caution is warranted. I undertake this task by first summarizing and contrasting several principal soteriological and eschatological tenets of transhumanism and Christianity, respectively, and then by arguing that the convictions underlying transhumanism are both inadequate and dangerous.

Being Saved from Being Human

According to transhumanism, embodiment is the principal problem of the human condition. The body imposes severe and intolerable limitations upon what humans can do and upon what they aspire to be. The body, for instance, constrains the will. A person cannot do everything he or she might want; not just anyone can be a professional athlete or the proverbial rocket scientist. More troubling, the body is a source of pain and suffering. As embodied beings humans are fragile and vulnerable; they can be injured or become ill. More depressingly, even if a person is fortunate enough to avoid any serious injuries or diseases, he or she is allotted only a limited amount of time. Embodied beings grow old and die. In short, human beings must be saved from their finite and mortal bodies.

The salvific response to this terrible plight is to wage a medical and technological war against aging and death. In the words of Max More, a leading transhumanist proponent, "Aging and death victimize all humans," thereby placing an unacceptable "imposition on the human race." Consequently, the "technological conquest of aging and death stands out as the most urgent, vital, worthy quest of our time."[3] Aging and death, then, should be regarded as diseases to be treated and eventually cured. Through a combination of anticipated advances in biotechnology, regenerative medicine, genetic manipulation, nanotechnology, bionics, and computer science, aging can presumably be arrested while humans simultaneously maintain or enhance their physical and cognitive performance. Individuals are thus enabled to live healthy, happy, productive, and long lives—perhaps very long or even endless ones. Evolution has, through natural selection, bequeathed to *Homo sapiens* bodies that serve as poor hosts for the information that constitutes their personalities (what the ancients called the soul, and moderns the will), and technological development and ingenuity can be used to negate, or eventually escape, the finite and mortal constraints that nature has imposed.

If humans are to be saved from their bodies, then ultimately death must also be conquered—dying must become a choice rather than a necessity. Through technology humans can transform themselves into a superior, and perhaps immortal, posthuman species. Although, as noted above, there is nothing new about a desire for immortality, the transhumanists are undertaking a unique quest for personal immortality. They are not endeavoring to live on after they die through a lineage, empire, or history, but to avoid death for a greatly extended period of time if not altogether. In undertaking this ambitious enterprise, however, the transhumanists are seemingly crashing against the insurmountable constraints of human biology. About 120 years appears to be the maximum amount of time that a human being can live. As Leonard Hayflick discovered, cellular division and replication in noncancerous cells can only occur a limited number of times. With each sequence, the telomeres on the DNA of each cell shorten. As the telomeres become shorter, they also become less efficient in replicating themselves. Eventually, the telomeres become so short that they can no longer function at all. This imperfect replication process also grows increasingly susceptible to mutations over time, leading to various diseases and the degeneration associated with aging. Consequently, the quest for personal immortality appears hopeless, for evolution has apparently destined human chromosomes to grow old and die.

Escape from the Jelly

The transhuman strategy for correcting this unfortunate problem is to develop technologies that can either reprogram or bypass the mortal limits of human DNA. Three prevalent and interrelated approaches are taken to achieve this goal. The first approach may be characterized as *biological immortality*. Some scientists believe that with anticipated developments in genetic and biotechnologies, the average life span can be increased dramatically, if not indefinitely. The twofold challenge is to prevent the shortening of the telomeres, and to ensure that degenerative mutations do not occur in cellar replication and rejuvenation. In addition, the immune system will be genetically enhanced and deleterious genetic defects will be removed or corrected to protect individuals from life-threatening and chronic diseases or disabilities.

Aubrey de Grey, for instance, contends that living for 150 or 200 years will soon become routine. With further technological innovation much more dramatic increases will be forthcoming, and immortality is not out of the question because infinite cellar rejuvenation cannot be ruled out in principle. For de Grey, winning the war against aging, and therefore death, is a matter of complex engineering. The DNA that natural selection haphazardly concocted and imposed upon humans simply needs to be redesigned in line with human values and purposes. Moreover, there is a moral imperative driving de Grey's quest for biological immortality, for he insists that mortality is not simply an unfortunate aspect of being human but is also an unmitigated tragedy that can and should be overcome through appropriate research and technological development.[4]

If, however, human biology proves less pliable than hoped—if, for instance, the Hayflick limit can only be extended modestly—all is still not lost in the war against aging and death. This leads to the second approach: *bionic immortality*. With anticipated advances in nanotechnology and robotics, as various body parts wear out they will be replaced with artificial substitutes. Synthetic blood vessels and skin could replace their less durable natural counterparts, and as muscles deteriorate, arms and legs will be assisted or replaced with sophisticated prosthetics. Nanobots will be injected to surgically repair or replace diseased organs, and neuroenhancers will be inserted into the brain to prevent the deterioration of memory and other cognitive functions. Admittedly, these artificial substitutes will also wear out over time, but they will be replaced with new and improved versions. Presumably, such maintenance could be undertaken indefinitely; in principle a bionic being could live forever, as long as its artificial parts are properly maintained, repaired, and replaced as needed. Additionally, physical and cognitive functions will not only be preserved but also enhanced. Individuals will enjoy the benefits of improved cardiovascular systems, greater strength and agility, and enhanced intelligence and recall.

Unfortunately, some liabilities accompany this bionic approach. The various electronic and mechanical systems can suffer serious malfunctions, and a hybrid host is still vulnerable to accidents or malicious acts resulting in death. Although a predominantly artificial body is an improvement over what nature offers, it is still not an ideal solution in overcoming finite and mortal limits. This leads us to the third, and most speculative, approach: *virtual immortality*. Leaders in the fields of artificial intelligence and robotics such as Ray Kurzweil and Hans Moravec argue that the information contained in the brain constituting a person's memories, experience, and personality can be digitized.[5] Therefore, in the near future, highly sophisticated imaging devices will scan the brain to collect this information and in turn upload it into a computer. Once this information has been organized and stored, it can then be downloaded into a robotic or virtual reality host. With frequently updated and multiple backups, the uploading and downloading process can be repeated indefinitely. Consequently, one's virtual self can be virtually immortal.

It may be objected that humans cannot be reduced to a series of zeros and ones and ones and zeros that can be shuffled about between robotic bodies and virtual reality programs. But Kurzweil and Moravec are quick to reply that because the mind is not a material object, and the mind is ultimately who and what a person is, then it cannot be anything other than information.

A personality comprises patterns of organized information that are formed and preserved over time. A biological body is merely a natural prosthetic hosting these patterns. Unfortunately, nature has not produced a very reliable or enduring prosthetic, so technology must be used to produce a better model. In liberating the mind from the biological body, nothing essential is lost—for if the information patterns of a person's identity are preserved, then, in Moravec's words, "I am preserved. The rest is mere jelly."[6] In short, technology can and should be developed to save individuals from the poor, jelly-like conditions of being human.

For the transhumanists, human biology, and its inherent finitude and mortality, is the enemy that must be conquered. The biological body is too fragile and limited to allow the full development of the mind's potential. A more congenial host must be constructed that provides the necessary time and augmentation enabling this development. Although the transhumanists reject a religious notion of a fall from which humans must be redeemed, they nonetheless offer a salvific and eschatological story. Through natural selection evolution has formed a species in which the mind is the most distinguishing trait. Yet humans remain hampered by severe biological limitations, as witnessed by their finitude and mortality. If the mind is to survive and flourish, if a person is to be saved from his or her body, then humans must take control of their evolutionary future by transforming themselves into a superior posthuman species.

The Paradox of Saving the Self

The urgency of this salvific story is seen in More's "Technological Self-Transformation."[7] According to More, "Life is fundamentally a ceaseless process, whose quintessence is a self-overcoming, a progression, a self-transformation and self-augmentation." More expansively, the chief characteristic of human life is a "perpetual drive toward its own increase and excellence." It is not coincidental that this drive is accompanied by an innate "desire for extreme longevity and the quest for physical immortality," because they constitute the prerequisites for maximum self-fulfillment. Although technology provides the practical means for achieving extreme longevity and immortality, more important, it enhances human autonomy by displacing the constraints of DNA, religion, political ideologies, and outdated social mores. Consequently, humans must "ignore the biological fundamentalists who will invoke 'God's plan' or 'the natural order of things,' in an effort to imprison us at the human level." Humans should instead accept the challenge of recreating themselves in their own image. But what is this image? According to More, there is no single correct answer. Because different individuals have

varying goals, "self-transformation is best implemented by creating for ourselves a paradigm, and idealised model of the person we want to become."
What More calls the "ideal self" or "Optimal Persona" is subject to periodic
review, assessment, and readjustment in order that the "higher being existing within us" will be realized.

As we shall see, More's salvific scheme is quixotic. He contends that
human evolution is driven by a desire for self-enhancement. To a limited
extent this is true given the tenets of evolutionary psychology. In the past,
however, this augmentation has been intergenerational, achieved incremen-
tally through the less invasive means of natural selection in tandem with
socialization. Biological and cultural evolution has been driven by the quality of the species rather than its individual members. But what More is proposing is a radical and rapid transformation of individuals rather than the
gradual improvement of the species. Furthermore, he assumes that such
technological self-transformation can be pursued without any correspond-
ing loss of subjectivity. This assumption, however, ignores the fact that the
mind evolved in conjunction with the brain, and more broadly the body.
There is, at best, scant evidence indicating what kind of subjectivity would
result if this linkage between mind and body were to be reconfigured or
eliminated.

Moreover, even if the kind of self-transformation More proposes proves
feasible, what exactly is his ideal self or Optimal Persona? He believes that
individuals can refashion themselves into the kind of beings they want to
become, but his proposed project of rational self-creation fails him because
of the libertarian rhetoric in which his rationality is embedded. His ideal self
exemplifies the autonomous individual, which means that he is appealing to
a historically conditioned tradition rather than any so-called pure rationality.
The eventual posthuman, then, is little more than a hyperlibertarian. What
More's salvific account demonstrates is the uneasy tension between his libertarian anthropology and posthuman eschatology.

More tries to resolve this tension by baldly asserting that the "Optimal
Persona is Nietzsche's *Übermensch*, the higher being existing within us as
potential waiting to be actualized." What would be some of the chief characteristics of this technologically constructed *Übermensch*? Despite More's
insistence that this latent potential can be actualized, he offers few sugges-
tions regarding what a world populated by Optimal Personae might be like.
We may turn to Hans Moravec, however, to gain a speculative glimpse of
the posthuman future. Moravec chronicles developments in computer science, artificial intelligence, and robotics during the second half of the twentieth century, and he describes anticipated advances in the next few decades.
Machines that are both intelligent and conscious will emerge by the middle

of the twenty-first century. Once this threshold is crossed, artificial life will evolve exponentially.[8] For humans to take full advantage of this technological breakthrough, they will need to merge with their "mind children." Eventually artificial life will evolve into pure thought, transforming the universe into an expanding cyberspace of pure mind.[9] Once this "Omega Point" has been reached, the resulting posthumans will be far removed from their human ancestors; they will become unrecognizable and incomprehensible from our current vantage point, but the subjective experiences of a primitive past need not be lost because "resurrection may be possible through the use of immense simulators."[10]

If Moravec's posthuman future is at all representative of transhumanist thought, then More's appeal to Nietzsche's *Übermensch* creates a greater problem than it solves. According to Nietzsche, nihilists will pave the way for the ascendant *Übermensch*. Nihilists will come to love rather than despise their mortal fate, enabling them to renounce any right to vengeance or dominating others. For Nietzsche, the only—admittedly thin—hope is that the nobility of the *Übermensch* will overcome the destructive *"resentiment"* of the last men. But what More fails to acknowledge is that the inspiration for a noble love of fate comes from the classic Greek philosophical embrace of suffering and tragedy. The *Übermensch* will presumably come to love the tragic fate of their mortality and the suffering that this love necessarily entails. But it is precisely this fate and its attendant misery that the transhumanists are trying to avoid. Consequently, they are not so much using technology to coax out the latent *Übermensch* as to create an entirely new species.

Yet if this is the case, is transhumanism simply a nihilistic expression of a technophilia devoid of any genuine love of fate? For if the nobility of mortality and suffering cannot be embraced, is there anything noble left to will? Rather, are they not attempting to abolish this fate by effectively willing the death of humankind? The only plausible salvific answer that transhumanism can offer is that humans must be saved from their finite and mortal bodies in order to perfect the latent qualities of their minds, and that this salvific strategy is in turn driven by an eschatological imperative to achieve this perfection through the creation of a superior posthuman species that can serve as a more enduring host for the information constituting one's being and identity. In short, the transhumanists wish to replace finitude and mortality with endless time as the definitive feature of the (post)human condition. But is this a salvific strategy and eschatological horizon that should be embraced?

What Must I Do to Be Saved?

Christian theology cannot embrace the transhumanist salvific strategy and eschatological horizon for reasons that are similar to its earlier rejection of the Manichean and Pelagian heresies. Transhumanism echoes a Manichean disdain of a corrupt, if not evil, material body from which the soul must be rescued. Yet for the transhumanists, unlike their ancient predecessors, the solution is not found in the release of death but in denying it by overcoming the finite and mortal limits of the body. There is also the Pelagian reiteration of the ability of humans to will themselves to perfection. The posthuman personifies the desire of the will to become the perfect being that it wills itself to be.

What is worrying for Christian theology is not that these old heresies have found a new voice but the disquieting moral beliefs accompanying them. The Manichean cannot resist hating the body, for it is a prison incarcerating the soul or will. The resulting aggravation, however, is not limited to self-loathing but is extended to a latent contempt of embodiment in general. If the body is merely the soul's prison or a poorly designed prosthesis of the will, then it is easier to justify physical neglect and abuse. The Pelagian quest for perfection cannot ultimately tolerate the imperfect. Regardless how perfection might be defined—for example, as a perfect body, soul, or will—that which remains imperfect or lacks the capability of being perfected should be eliminated or prevented. Alarmingly, Pelagians of every age often appeal to medical rhetoric to achieve the perfection they envision.[11] Is it not a concern for public hygiene that inspires eugenic programs to sanitize the race and to inhibit the birth of those who would infect it? If the posthuman exemplifies the triumph of the will, then there is an accompanying and inescapable logic of the necessity of eliminating or preventing that which is judged to stand in the way of its final and perfect culmination.

These criticisms do not suggest that the transhumanists endorse cruelty and intolerance. Rather, old heresies in new garb serve as reminders that good intentions alone cannot prevent unintended yet nevertheless evil consequences. The problem with heresy is not that it deliberately advocates what is wrong, but that it elevates half-truths to the whole truth, thereby distorting the good that it is purportedly seeking to achieve. According to Hannah Arendt, it is thoughtlessness instead of malice that results in evil acts that are banal rather than malicious.[12] In rebutting these heresies, Christian theology has appealed to the goodness of the body and more expansively to the good of embodiment. The particular challenge in response to transhumanism, therefore, is not to remain human but to remain creaturely, which by definition is to be finite and mortal, and therefore inescapably embodied. It is in and through their bodies that human creatures give and receive life, and in and through their bodies that they are in fellowship with one another and with their Creator.

This affirmation of embodiment is derived from the doctrine of the Incarnation. Through the Incarnation, God vindicates and redeems the creation from its futility, thereby conquering death as witnessed by the resurrection of Jesus Christ from the dead. It is the empty tomb that most starkly differentiates Christian eschatology from its posthuman counterpart. The soul (or the information constituting one's personality) is not rescued from the body, but rather it is as an embodied creature that one is redeemed by God. The doctrine of Christ's bodily resurrection, therefore, should not be casually discarded as a relic of a credulous age, for it serves as a powerful reminder that the body is God's good gift and not something to be despised. Christians affirm the credo that the resurrection of the body is part of their destiny of eternal fellowship with the triune God. For Christians, death is a real fate, but it is not to be either feared or loved, for in Christ death it has already been overcome and redeemed within eternity.

Consequently, what separates Christian from posthuman eschatology is that the latter seeks immortality while the former awaits eternity. Transformation does not consist of greatly extended longevity culminating in virtual immortality, but of a temporal finitude and mortality that have already been transcended by eternity. It is the finitude and mortality of being human and human being that are affirmed by the Incarnation. This is not a condition from which creatures need rescuing, for it is only as finite and mortal creatures that they are saved. To denigrate the body is to deny the very grace that sustains, vindicates, and redeems the human condition. It is the Word made flesh and not flesh transformed into data that is ultimately salvific.

Dying to Live

Ironically, in their quest for extreme longevity and immortality the transhumanists become fixated upon mortality, and it is a perilous, if not deadly, fixation. According to Arendt, birth and death are the two definitive conditions demarcating the human condition.[13] It is pursuing the former rather than avoiding the latter, however, that should provide the principal metaphor for ordering human life and lives. Natality ensures a generational continuity over time, while also encapsulating the possibility for change and improvement. Each new birth simultaneously embodies a continuous line of memory and anticipation, a self-giving that creates a recipient who is both like and yet unlike the giver. The gift of every parent is also the unique possibility of each child.

Although death is not something to be embraced lovingly, mortality is not humankind's great curse. When death is perceived as nothing more than a cruel fate, natality is robbed of its power to renew and regenerate. To be fixated on mortality is to promote a social and political order that attempts to cheat that fate for as long as possible. Survival becomes *the* consuming desire that in turn corrupts all other values and considerations. The birth of a child holds no hope or promise, but serves only as a reminder of a mortal fate to be despised and despaired. Consequently, replication—as opposed to reproduction or procreation—becomes the tyrannous rationale of personal survival pervading all resulting relationships and associations.

It is telling that the transhumanists have little to say substantively about natality and mortality. Ranting against death as a tragedy reveals nothing other than emotive pique. At best, mortality becomes an *is* from which the *ought* of its negation is derived. Yet the ensuing imperative can only be achieved by relentlessly seeking the destruction of the finite and mortal qualities that make its formulation possible. Is the surgical removal of humankind's creaturely ontology really the only advice that the transhumanists have to offer in the face of death? If so, then the underlying survivalist ethic becomes more explicable, helping to account for an equally vacuous understanding of natality. More often than not, the transhumanists simply ignore any intergenerational questions in order to concentrate on the more pressing question of extending personal longevity.

This lack of serious engagement with the moral, social, and political significance of natality amplifies the transhumanists' morbid fascination with mortality. If the only meaningful way to contend against the old enemy of death is for one to survive for as long as possible, then it is absurd to contemplate any tasks of social and political reproduction. There are simply no corporate institutions or structures requiring continuity, renewal, and unanticipated possibility, for the future is merely a self-absorbing extension and projection of the present. Yet to ignore or denigrate the significance of natality is to reject the underlying unity and equality that both binds and liberates generations over time. To displace this with survivalist engineering is to succumb to the tyranny of the present over the future. It is to enthrone the self-maker over the future self, the creator over the artifact, for the latter can never be genuinely free from the originating intentions of the former. The *made* cannot share fully the equal fellowship of the *begotten*.[14] Ironically, as one attempts to transform oneself into a superior being, the resulting posthuman becomes enslaved to itself as a self-constructed artifact, a semblance of a semblance.

Francis Fukuyama is right in insisting that although transhumanism may look like a silly cult, it is nonetheless a dangerous idea, for it is essentially an idolatrous religion proffering a counterfeit salvation.[15] It is counterfeit because of its inability to see finitude and mortality as anything more than unwanted constraints upon the will to be conquered and discarded. But the cost of such a victory is the elimination of the very creatures that need to be saved. One has to destroy humankind in order to save human beings.

Despite all the survival and immortality rhetoric, at its core transhumanism is a religion predicated upon a death wish. And even if none of the envisioned technological developments come true, it remains a dangerous idea, for it exemplifies and amplifies the technological and nihilistic ontology of late modernity in which the creation and its creatures are subjected to an endless and violent process of construction, deconstruction, and reconstruction. Transhumanism is a dangerous idea not because of its futuristic orientation but because its rhetoric is hyperbolic commentary on our present circumstances.

As N. Katherine Hayles has observed, "People become posthuman because they think they are posthuman."[16] What, then, happens to the moral and religious imagination when such posthumans view embodiment as an enemy to be despised and warred against rather than a definitive feature of a creature bearing the *imago Dei*? This is not to say that finitude and mortality are inherently good, for they are admittedly the source of pain, suffering, and ultimately death. Yet it is a necessary feature of being a creature that has been created by a good God. It is precisely in being finite and mortal that humans are reminded that they are creatures created by a creator, and not self-made artifacts. In consenting to the necessity of death, they affirm the goodness of the One who created them. And remaining creaturely as they await their redemption is a good well worth defending, a good that should inform a theological and moral imagination that claims to be Christian.

Notes

1. On "object of faith," see Niebuhr, *Radical Monotheism*, 119–22. On "ultimate concern," see Tillich, *Dynamics of Faith*, 1–29.

2. Teilhard de Chardin, *Future of Man*; Hefner, *Technology*, 73–88.

3. More, "On Becoming Posthuman."

4. See, e.g., de Grey, "Strategies for Engineered Negligible Senescence"; and de Grey, "War on Aging."

5. See Kurzweil, *Age of Spiritual Machines*; and Kurzweil, *Singularity*. And see Moravec, *Mind Children*; and Moravec, *Robot*.

6. Moravec, *Mind Children*, 117.

7. More, "Technological Self-Transformation."

8. See Moravec, *Robot*, 15–126.

9. Ibid., 163–89.

10. Ibid., 201–2; Moravec, *Mind Children*, 123.

11. See Passmore, *Perfectibility of Man*.

12. See Arendt, *Eichmann in Jerusalem*.

13. Arendt, *Human Condition*, 7–11.

14. This distinction between making and begetting and the resulting inequality between the maker and the made as opposed to the underlying equality of

the begetter and the begotten is derived from Oliver O'Donovan's moral and theological analysis of reproductive technology; see, O'Donovan, *Begotten or Made?*
  15. Fukuyama, "World's Most Dangerous Ideas: Transhumanism."
  16. Hayles, *How We Became Posthuman*, 6.

References

Arendt, Hannah. *Eichmann in Jerusalem: A Report on the Banality of Evil.* New York: Penguin Books, 1992.

———. *The Human Condition.* Chicago: University of Chicago Press, 1998.

Saint Augustine. *Concerning the City of God against the Pagans*, translated by Henry Bettenson. London: Penguin Books, 1984.

Fukuyama, Francis. "The World's Most Dangerous Ideas: Transhumanism." *Foreign Policy* 144 (2004): 42–43.

de Grey, Aubrey, ed. "Strategies for Engineered Negligible Senescence: Why Genuine Control of Aging May Be Foreseeable." *Annals of the New York Academy of Science* 1019 (June 2004): xv–xvi, 1–592.

———. "The War on Aging." In *The Scientific Conquest of Death*, edited by Immortality Institute. Buenos Aires: Libros EnRed, 2004.

Hayles, N. Katherine. *How We Became Posthuman: Virtual Bodies in Cybernetics, Literature, and Informatics.* Chicago: University of Chicago Press, 1999.

Hefner, Philip. *Technology and Human Becoming.* Minneapolis: Fortress Press, 2003.

Kurzweil, Ray. *The Age of Spiritual Machines: When Computers Exceed Human Intelligence.* New York: Penguin Books, 2000.

———. *The Singularity Is Near: When Humans Transcend Biology.* New York: Penguin Books, 2005.

Moravec, Hans. *Mind Children: The Future of Robot and Human Intelligence.* Cambridge, MA: Harvard University Press, 1988.

———. *Robot. Mere Machines to Transcendent Mind.* Oxford: Oxford University Press, 1999.

More, Max. "On Becoming Posthuman." www.maxmore.com/becoming.htm.

———. "Technological Self-Transformation." www.maxmore.com/selftrns.htm.

Niebuhr, H. Richard. *Radical Monotheism and Western Culture.* Louisville: Westminster / John Knox Press, 1993.

O'Donovan, Oliver. *Begotten or Made?* Oxford: Clarendon Press, 1984.

Passmore, John. *The Perfectibility of Man.* New York: Charles Scribner's Sons, 1970.

Teilhard de Chardin, Pierre. *The Future of Man*, translated by Norman Denny. London: Collins, 1964.

Tillich, Paul. *Dynamics of Faith.* New York: Harper & Row, 1957.

Chapter Twelve

Transcendence, Technological Enhancement, and Christian Theology

GERALD MCKENNY

In an essay published in 2004 Francis Fukuyama famously (or for some, notoriously) identified transhumanism as "the world's most dangerous idea."[1] Many Christians would agree with Fukuyama's condemnation of any program that has as its goal, or at least as a welcome prospect, the transformation of humans into "future beings whose basic capacities so radically exceed those of present humans as to be no longer unambiguously human by our current standards."[2] Christians who share Fukuyama's concern often align themselves with a position, prominently represented on the President's Council on Bioethics during the administration of George W. Bush, that is often suspicious of robust forms of transcendence.

The topic of transhumanism and transcendence is therefore an apt one for Christian theology. In this chapter I argue that a proper Christian approach to the prospect of human technological enhancement should, in partial opposition to Fukuyama and others who share his position, acknowledge the legitimacy of some degree of dissatisfaction with the limits of human nature as it is but should not confuse a Christian conception of transcendence with a transhumanist one.

The Dilemma of Transcendence

In *A Secular Age* the philosopher Charles Taylor discusses a central dilemma faced by reflective people in modern Western societies. On the one hand, the moral self-understanding of these societies is strongly marked by the critique of certain forms of transcendence that originated in the premodern West. According to one version of the modern critique, traditional Christianity denigrates ordinary human desires and fulfillments, valorizing their renunciation in favor of the love of God. According to another version, which has found an eloquent voice in Martha Nussbaum, Western culture has been marked by the aspiration to transcend human vulnerabilities, neediness, and particular attachments, promoting the ideal of a life that is free of these limitations. In both cases, it is argued, the aspiration to transcendence diminishes our humanity and diverts us from the pursuit of properly human goods. A genuinely human life, so the argument goes, would seek meaning and fulfillment in ordinary attachments and attainments conditioned by our finitude, vulnerability, and bodily nature rather than attempting to renounce or overcome these characteristics and limitations.

On the other hand, Taylor argues, the refusal of every aspiration to transcendence also seems to diminish us. Indeed, modernity itself is as strongly marked by its own forms of transcendence as it is by its critiques of transcendence. Love that extends beyond erotic attachment to embrace a universal concern, the disciplining of tendencies to aggression and violence, and forms of self-overcoming promoted by thinkers such as Nietzsche and Foucault are all characteristic features of modern ethical life. It is difficult, Taylor asserts, to imagine how a life devoid of these or some other forms of transcendence could be genuinely fulfilling.[3]

Two especially salient points emerge from Taylor's account. First, modernity is not characterized by a rejection of transcendence in favor of immanence, which would mean, in this context, a life lived entirely within the horizon of ordinary desires and natural ends. Aspirations to transcendence do not disappear but take new forms in the face of the critique of previous forms (even as these older forms of transcendence persist). As Taylor implicitly suggests, this is apparent in the case of Nietzsche, who is at once the most vociferous critic of what he sees as Christian transcendence of the body and sensual desire and the great exhorter to self-overcoming. Second, this modern condition poses an ongoing problem for modern people because it is by no means easy to draw the line between those aspirations to transcendence that diminish us and those without which our lives would be impoverished.

Taylor's discussion of ordinary human life and its transcendence focuses almost exclusively on ethical activity and social reform, omitting the role of technology in modern forms of transcendence. Yet one of the most significant sites for the enactment of the dilemma he describes is technological enhancement. (By technological enhancement I mean the use of technologies such as genetic engineering, psychopharmacology, nanotechnology, information technology, and neural interface technology, among others, to alter human characteristics.) On the one side are transhumanists such as Nick Bostrom, James Hughes, and Ray Kurzweil (or, reaching further back, Julian Huxley and Pierre Teilhard de Chardin) who, in the words of the organization Humanity+ (formerly known as the World Transhumanist Association), hold "that the human species in its current form does not represent the end of our development but rather a comparatively early phase" and who support, at least in principle, the overcoming of human limitations and

vulnerabilities.[4] On the other side are what we might call humanistic naturalists such as Francis Fukuyama, Leon Kass, and Michael Sandel (or, reaching
further back, Hannah Arendt and Hans Jonas) who, despite their differences,
hold that (in the terms Jonas urged against Ernst Bloch) "humanity as it is,"
is an objective good that demands our respect.[5] Humanity is not something
still to be "realized" by technological reshaping but finds its worth or dignity
in its finite, vulnerable, embodied nature—that is, in precisely those features
that transhumanists hope to alter or transcend.

The debate between transhumanism and humanistic naturalism is fundamentally a debate about the good. The issue at stake is what constitutes or
would constitute true fulfillment or flourishing. As such, this debate seems
to illustrate in an especially poignant way the dilemma Taylor describes: We
find in it the critique of transcendence and the valuation of human life in its
vulnerability and neediness, the aspiration to a distinctively modern form
of transcendence in the removal of these natural limitations, and, given
the inextricability of technology from our lives, the difficulty—even for the
humanistic naturalists insofar as they do not reject human enhancement
in toto—of determining which aspirations to transcendence fulfill us and
which diminish us.

Transcendence, Immanence, and Human Fulfillment

Before we explore this dilemma as it arises in the relation of Christianity to transhumanism and humanistic naturalism, two preliminary points
are in order. The first point has to do with the relationship between transhumanism and humanistic naturalism on the one side and transcendence
and immanence on the other side. It is tempting to characterize the issue
of the debate in a way that identifies transhumanism with transcendence
and humanistic naturalism with immanence. Transhumanists, after all, treat
human nature in its present form as merely a transitional stage to a posthuman reality, or at least many of them do. And humanistic naturalists, as I
have just noted, argue for leaving human nature as it is and finding value or
dignity in its limitations and vulnerability. If the aspiration to transcendence
implies that the end at which our activities should aim is found in a state that
goes beyond our present limitations, then transhumanism would fall on the
side of transcendence and humanistic naturalism on the side of immanence.
Yet we will see that the matter is more complicated than this simple distinction suggests.

One factor that complicates this simple distinction is that at least some
versions of humanistic naturalism propound their own version of transcendence, arguing that it is in and through our natural limitations, and not apart

from them, that we may experience a kind of transcendence that is essential to genuine fulfillment. Nussbaum refers to this form of transcendence as "internal" transcendence, distinguishing it from "external" transcendence, which is the aspiration to a life that is free of vulnerability, neediness, and other conditions of finitude. She includes under this heading the depth and richness of perception and responsiveness that she finds in writers such as Henry James and Marcel Proust, which bring one to a more profound understanding of and engagement with the world, and the desire to leave a lasting mark on the world through one's deeds or works. Kass appeals to a similar yet far less snobbish conception of transcendence when he explores the complex interweaving of sameness and otherness, mortality and permanence, and self-regard and other-regard that he takes to be the meaning of human sexual reproduction.[6]

Furthermore, when transhumanism is stripped of its often overblown rhetoric, it often amounts to the realization in a posthuman (or altered human) form of the very ideal that motivated the modern turn from transcendence to immanence—namely, the attainment of a state in which humans would enjoy greater longevity, freedom from suffering and disease, and increased cognitive capacities. Transhumanist lists of desired capabilities and states exhibit a remarkable continuity with those of Bacon, Descartes, and other paradigmatically modern thinkers who sought to direct the pursuit of knowledge from theoretical contemplation to the improvement of ordinary life.[7] It is true that at some indeterminable point the line is crossed that separates improvement of this life and an altogether different sort of life, and the turn to immanence itself becomes a return to transcendence. I argue below that transhumanism is ultimately committed to such a move. It is also true that the value transhumanists place on radically enhanced capacities and their correlate goods typically goes well beyond what such capacities and goods would allegedly do for ordinary life. But it is important to keep in mind that it begins with aims that are continuous with those of early modern champions of immanence. If some forms of Western asceticism attempt to attain a transcendent end in part through the renunciation of immanent goods, transhumanism begins with the attempt to attain immanent goods through the transcendence of natural human limitations. To identify transhumanism with transcendence and humanistic naturalism with immanence is therefore a gross oversimplification.[8]

The second preliminary point has to do with deciding who counts as a transhumanist or a humanistic naturalist, and on what grounds. This is not the place for anything like a rigorous definition or set of criteria for inclusion and exclusion, but it is important to distinguish a transhumanist, for whom transition to a higher form of humanity or to a posthuman form seems to be regarded as good in itself, at least in principle, from a utilitarian, for whom such a transition may simply be accepted as the cumulative result of efforts to promote aggregate welfare, just as it is important to distinguish a humanistic naturalist, for whom worth or dignity is inseparable from natural vulnerabilities and limitations, from someone for whom moral norms constrain what can be rightly done to overcome these vulnerabilities and limitations but who does not object in principle to their overcoming.

As an example of the first distinction, John Harris argues with regard to potential population-level changes to human beings that "if the gains were important enough (sufficiently beneficial) and the risks acceptable, we would want to make the relevant alterations and be justified in so doing, indeed . . . would have an obligation to make such changes." But this is all, morally speaking, that is at stake in the matter; "whether any proposed changes amount to changes in human nature, or involve further evolution, seems ethically uninteresting."[9] A transhumanist, conversely, is someone for whom the prospect of changes in human nature or the continuation of evolution is not ethically uninteresting, for whom the very prospect of higher stages of development of humanity exercises at least some normative pull, even if the desirability of the states and capabilities themselves (e.g., freedom from disease or enhanced cognitive capacity) offer a sufficient motive.[10] With regard to the second distinction, it is possible to argue that the means whereby human enhancement would be pursued are morally wrong—for example, that genetic interventions on embryos or gametes would violate the autonomy of the child or future child, impose unjustifiable risks, or erode the grounds of equality—without arguing that the end itself (i.e., the improvement of human nature) is wrong. Jürgen Habermas is one among many critics of human enhancement who opposes it on grounds such as these.[11]

These preliminary points allow us to identify and isolate an issue that is of interest to Christian theology but is often obscured in debates over the technological enhancement of humans. The issue does not simply pit the case for transcendence against the case for immanence. Nor is it simply a debate over whether we should proceed with the technological enhancement of humans. Rather, the issue is whether genuine fulfillment is to be found in a life that is needy, mortal, vulnerable to disease and disability, bound by conditions of embodiment, and limited to the kinds of transcendence we are capable of experiencing through our finite, bodily nature and not apart from it; or whether it is to be found in release from at least many of these limitations in order to live as long as we want, free from bodily affliction and physical and mental decline and able to exercise control over our moods and thoughts, to experience new forms of consciousness and sensation, and so on. Transhumanists and humanistic naturalists may not be at the center of debates over the ethics of human enhancement, which most often are carried out by adherents of the positions from which we distinguished transhumanists and humanistic naturalists in the previous paragraph. And it is likely, given the forms and practices of bioethical debate, that the ethical and regulatory regimes that govern human enhancement will be decided by the adherents of those other positions and not by the transhumanists and humanistic naturalists. But this does not mean that the latter do not understand more deeply than the former what is morally and spiritually at stake in human enhancement.

Christian Transcendence and Humanistic Naturalism

Although the transhumanists and humanistic naturalists understand in a profound way what is ultimately at stake in human technological enhancement, it can be argued from a Christian theological standpoint that neither of them gets it quite right. The most intractable problems with humanistic naturalism have to do with the difficulty it has allowing for legitimate dissatisfaction with the limitations of human nature as we experience it. The point is not that humanistic naturalists argue for leaving everything just as it is. They are sometimes accused of rejecting human biotechnology altogether, but the charge is false. Still, humanistic naturalists do seem to face a difficulty in cases of biomedical technologies that enjoy widespread acceptance but would seem to be suspect from a perspective that accords normative status to unaltered human nature. Must humanistic naturalists reject mood-altering drugs, genetic therapies, and even vaccines? Do they regret the developments that have greatly expanded life expectancy in the past century? The answer to all these questions is negative.[12] Humanistic naturalists are usually quick to distinguish the prevention and treatment of disease and restoration of function, on the one hand, from enhancement of human traits and capabilities, on the other hand, and to argue that their critiques of human biotechnology apply only to the latter.[13]

But the distinction between therapy and enhancement is a notoriously problematic one. In the first place, it is not always clear whether a condition being treated is a disease or a trait (think of the controversies over the diagnosis of attention deficit hyperactivity disorder). Humanistic naturalists acknowledge that this distinction can be difficult to make in practice. But even where this difference can be made clear, it is often difficult to say why the same drug can be legitimately used to treat a disease but not to alter a trait.[14] This kind of case does present a problem for humanistic naturalists, because it requires them to subordinate the relief of suffering to what seems, in the face of suffering, to be a rather abstract distinction between therapy and enhancement.

These problems faced by humanistic naturalists are widely recognized and have been discussed at length, so there is no need to dwell on them here.[15] The point in bringing them up is to show that their counsel to accept natural human limitations does not lead them to argue that everything should be left just as it is. Rather, the problem with humanistic naturalism is a much more fundamental and much less frequently discussed one: There are reasons for refusing to be satisfied with human nature within the horizon of its natural limitations, and at least some of these reasons have strong theological justifications. The point is not just that the vulnerabilities and limitations of human nature are at least as much a threat to genuine fulfillment as they are the ground of the latter. Humanistic naturalists can concede this point and can consistently argue that human beings should do all that they can, within moral and prudential constraints, to extend the life expectancy of individuals, eliminate diseases, fight the physical and mental decline that accompanies aging, and so forth.[16]

None of this kind of activity entails the aspirations to immortality with the immunity to suffering and perpetual youth and vigor that humanistic naturalists criticize. What humanistic naturalists cannot consistently hold, however, is that the highest human fulfillment exceeds what human beings can experience or bring about through their natural capacities and that the goods of finite human life must ultimately be understood in light of this ultimate fulfillment. To concede this would be to hold that external transcendence is necessary to human fulfillment and that the ethical and spiritual meanings that depend on limitation and vulnerability, including those meanings that constitute internal transcendence, ultimately lie in their relation to external transcendence. Yet if human fulfillment ultimately involves external transcendence, then there is sufficient reason for refusing to rest satisfied with human life as it is lived within the horizon of natural limitations and vulnerabilities. And if this is so, humanistic naturalism is an inadequate account of human fulfillment.

Christian theology is committed to the claim that human fulfillment entails external transcendence. Saint Augustine articulates the consensus of traditional Catholic, Orthodox, and Protestant theology when he repeatedly refers to the highest human good by quoting Psalm 73:28: "But for me it is good to cleave to God." Human fulfillment ultimately consists of communion with God. Yet to enjoy this fulfillment in its highest degree transcends natural human capacities; it is not fully attainable in this life and lies beyond what human beings are able to bring about by the exercise of these capacities. This basic point has, of course, been developed in many different ways.

But here, for purposes of economy, I consider how it is understood in the tradition of Thomas Aquinas, which has brought a high degree of precision of thought to it. Most of what I say also applies to many non-Thomistic forms of Christian theology; indeed, virtually nothing that I say about Aquinas could not have been said, albeit in a different way, by Karl Barth.[17] And though I prefer Barth's formulation to Aquinas's for various reasons, the fundamental role played in his account by Christology is difficult to make clear without a lengthy discussion. I therefore forgo whatever benefits follow from Barth's formulation for the more economical formulation of Aquinas. For Aquinas, the ultimate good is knowledge of God that participates in God's own self-knowledge. However, the human intellect is not capable of knowing God as God is in God's divine nature but requires for this knowledge a power of illumination that is given to it by God as a gift of grace. Though knowledge of God by human beings does not amount to a full comprehension of God even with this gift, and so the contrast between creature and Creator is never overcome, it is nevertheless genuine knowledge of God in God's own nature, and this knowledge is the highest human good.[18]

As Thomists understand it, then, the ultimate good is a good that exceeds natural human capacities and can be attained only by a gift of grace that extends these capacities beyond their natural capability. In this sense Thomism offers a version of external transcendence. It makes plausible, at least for many Christians, the notion of a good that can be enjoyed only by a radical extension or transformation of our natural capacities and that we who remain (for now, at least) bound by our natural limitations cannot adequately describe or even name but can only gesture toward. And anyone for whom the notion of such a good is plausible should be able to understand why some people, at least, are attracted to the transhumanist vision and find themselves dissatisfied with the counsel of humanistic naturalists to remain within the horizon of our natural limitations.

Christian Transcendence and Transhumanism

From the fact that Christian conceptions of the ultimate good entail external transcendence, however, it does not follow either that Christian theology should endorse the forms of external transcendence promoted by transhumanists or that humanistic naturalism has the wrong account of the ethics of human technological enhancement. In what follows I focus mostly on the first point. The Christian conception of external transcendence, at least in the Thomist version we have been considering, differs in significant ways from transhumanist versions. Ironically, transhumanists and humanistic naturalists are in agreement that the enjoyment of goods that transcend our natural human capacities must come at the cost of these capacities and therefore of our humanity. Both are convinced that external transcendence is incompatible with human nature as we now know it. It is just this assumption, however, that Christian theology rejects in its conception of communion with God. According to this conception, though natural human capacities are incapable of attaining this good, it is a good to which these capacities, and not some others, are suited.

Moreover, although these capacities must be extended in order to enjoy this good, it is the gift of divine grace that extends them, and not a technological enhancement of their natural capability or their transformation into some other capacities. Finally, although the ultimate good exceeds human capacities, it is still a human good, a good for humans, and the external transcendence made possible by divine grace, far from denigrating humanity, is what makes it possible to enjoy this good, which infinitely exceeds and overwhelms our capacities, while we remain human.[19]

For all these reasons it is a mistake to suppose that technological enhancement can bring anyone closer to this good by enhancing the natural capacities that share in it or by transforming them into something else. Indeed, if technological enhancement were to result in a radical transformation of human capacities—a transformation sufficiently radical to justify the label "posthuman"—the enjoyment of this good, at least in its highest form, might be foreclosed altogether. Communion with God, the ultimate good, is a good for which humans were created and equipped to enjoy. In this sense, at least, Christianity is unabashedly humanist.[20]

In contrast to the version of external transcendence found in Christianity (or at least in Thomist and other similar interpretations of Christianity), the version found in transhumanism separates the good from human nature as it is. This point is not immediately apparent, and it may not characterize all forms of transhumanist thought, but it seems to be entailed by the fundamental vision of transhumanism. It takes some effort, however, to see how this is so. Transhumanist conceptions of the good combine a Nietzschean sense of dismay at the thought that the human being might not become all that it is capable of becoming with a quasi-utilitarian commitment to the promotion of the good in abstraction from the question of whose good it is. Thus the "Transhumanist Declaration" begins with a human perspective, referring to the "the possibility of broadening of human potential" in its first article and going on to pronounce, in the second article, that "we believe that humanity's potential is still mostly unrealized."[21]

In his own way, of course, Nietzsche would concur. But the same organization that adopted this declaration distinguishes transhumanism from humanism by pointing out that whereas both are committed to the use of "rational means to improve the human condition and the external world," transhumanists are also committed to using such means to improve the human organism itself: "We can also use technological means that will eventually enable us to move beyond what some would think of as 'human.'"[22] At this point transhumanism departs from Nietzsche, who would have scorned any good that cannot be made intelligible as the result of human activity and that can be recognized as good only by abstracting from human desires. What could motivate us, Nietzsche would ask, to pursue such a good, except some debilitating form of human self-hatred?

It is not immediately obvious, however, that transhumanists abstract the good from human desires and wants. Transhumanists often refer to greater or more intense or lasting experiences of things that many or most humans currently consider to be good, such as knowledge of reality, aesthetic sensibility, and emotional breadth and depth, to name a few. Thus they note: "It seems likely," therefore, "that the simple fact of living an indefinitely long, healthy, active life would take anyone to posthumanity if they went on accumulating memories, skills, and intelligence."[23] Yet there is no doubt that at least some transhumanists seem to be committed to holding that future posthumans may have significantly or even entirely different ideas of what is good. However, even this commitment does not necessarily entail that these ideas of the good are unrelated to what humans now desire, value, or want. Nick Bostrom, drawing on David Lewis's dispositional theory of value, points out that the fact that there are goods greater than we can currently value does not imply that these goods are independent of what we currently value. It may simply be the case that we currently lack the capacities to grasp them fully—a lack that in the case of some such goods would presumably be overcome by enhancement of the relevant capacities. Thus, as Bostrom concludes, "the transhumanist view that we ought to explore the realm of posthuman values does not entail that we should forgo our current values. The posthuman values can be our current values, albeit ones that we have not yet clearly comprehended."[24]

However, Bostrom is arguing only that transhumanism does not *necessarily* entail a break with what we currently value. "Transhumanism," he claims in a more general programmatic statement, "promotes the quest to develop further so that we can explore hitherto inaccessible realms of value."[25] Some of these realms of value may be continuous with what we currently value. But Bostrom readily admits—and accepts—that some modifications of our capacities would likely constitute a change of identity. Such a change of identity, if it occurred, would undoubtedly entail the possibility that what our successors value will be discontinuous with what we value.

This brings us to the quasi-utilitarian nature of the transhumanist conception of the good, in which there is an obligation to promote the good as such, without regard to whose good it is. The problem is not only that the pursuit of such a good is in principle exercised at the expense of our humanity—a condition that Nietzsche, along with other humanistic naturalists, deplored and that Christianity, despite the criticisms to the contrary, never forces us into. Nor is the problem only that the prospect of a good that may be radically different from what we now recognize and value as good disqualifies all the efforts (no doubt sincere) of transhumanists to place technological enhancement in a modern moral framework committed to welfare, respect for autonomy and individual rights, and fairness—a framework that is patently dependent not only on human nature as it is but even on modern society as it is.[26] In addition to these very real issues, there is the problem that no account can be given of a good that has no relation to our human nature, and so the transhumanist conception of the good must necessarily be an empty one. In the end the good as transhumanists understand it can only be described as the unknown correlate of the radically enhanced human capacities that are capable of grasping it.[27] It follows that all transhumanists can do is urge us to keep pushing the technology further on the grounds that there will be great goods to enjoy—whether for us or, more likely, for our successors, whoever or whatever they are. And if not in principle then at least in practice, this seems inevitably to subordinate the pursuit of the good to the pursuit of power.

Conclusion

Such are the difficulties that we humans encounter when we separate the good from our human nature, and we can now see why Christians need not and should not endorse external transcendence as it is understood and promoted in transhumanist thought, any more than they should confine themselves to the internal transcendence described by humanistic naturalists. However, although Christian theology cannot be satisfied with internal transcendence, it does seem to be committed, in Jonas's terms, to the claim that "humanity as it is, is good." External transcendence in the tradition of Christian theology articulated by Thomism does not require or even permit the radical alteration of human nature because it is precisely this nature (and, as far as we know, only this nature) that grace grants participation in the ultimate good of communion with God in its highest form. In all its vulnerability, neediness, and finite limitation, and in spite of its corruption by sin, human nature is good, and is to be recognized and valued as such, because it is the being with this nature whom God has chosen to enjoy the highest form of communion with God. And this conviction brings Christian ethics closer to the humanistic naturalist view of the ethics of human enhancement than to the transhumanist view.

The life that God makes suitable for the highest form of communion with God is human life in all its neediness, vulnerability, and limitation. The aspiration to overcome these conditions, which technology may sooner or later be able to fulfill, at least to some degree, is therefore a misguided aspiration. However, it does not follow that it is ethically wrong in principle from a Christian point of view to seek not only to mitigate but also to eliminate certain effects of human vulnerability (e.g., susceptibility to diseases, premature death) or even to chip away at human limitations (e.g., by increasing cognitive capacities or the human life span). Efforts such as these do not necessarily express the aspiration to overcome the conditions of neediness, vulnerability, and limitation themselves. Of course, it is impossible to determine the precise point at which such efforts do express this aspiration. Moreover, these efforts may be ethically wrong or problematic for many reasons other than those having to do with this aspiration. For these reasons it would take a much longer chapter to sort out the ethics of technological enhancement that follows from the notion of external transcendence that I have ascribed to Christian theology. All I have sought to do here is to distinguish this form of transcendence from the forms found in humanistic naturalism and transhumanism, to argue that it is not subject to the criticisms of external transcendence made by humanistic naturalists, and to show how it avoids the problems of those forms of external transcendence found in transhumanist thought.

Notes

1. Fukuyama, "World's Most Dangerous Ideas: Transhumanism," 42–43.

2. Humanity+, "Transhumanist FAQ: What Is a Posthuman?" http://humanity plus.org/learn/transhumanist-faq/.

3. Taylor, *Secular Age*, 618–39. Taylor is in part responding to Nussbaum, "Transcending Humanity," 365–91, which itself is a response to Taylor, "Review Article on Martha Nussbaum."

4. Humanity+, "Transhumanist FAQ: What Is Transhumanism?" This definition leaves open the question of whether the later phases implied by it involve the alteration or further development of entities that remain human, the transformation of at least some humans into another biological species, or their transformation into some nonbiological form. The term "posthuman" tends to be used indiscriminately to refer to any or all of these alternatives.

5. Jonas, *Imperative of Responsibility*.

6. Nussbaum, "Transcending Humanity," 379–82; Kass, *Life, Liberty*, 153–57. Needless to say, this does not imply that Nussbaum agrees with Kass's use of this conception of transcendence and its ethical significance.

7. See Bostrom, "Transhumanist Values." Bostrom adds new or enhanced sensory capacities and control of moods but otherwise largely repeats the traditional list.

8. It is also a mistake to think of transhumanism as postmodern and humanistic naturalism as a throwback to the premodern. In its hope of attaining longevity, freedom from disease and suffering, and enhanced cognitive capacities transhumanism, as we have just seen, are only the latest versions of a modern dream with a long pedigree. For its part, humanistic naturalism, with its turn to ordinary life and its satisfaction with a minimally transcendent horizon, is itself thoroughly modern, despite strong antimodern strains in some of its chief expositors (e.g., Jonas and Kass).

9. Harris, *Enhancing Evolution*, 37. In the quoted material Harris is summarizing the argument of his previous book—Harris, *Wonderwoman and Superman*.

10. Some might argue that the normative pull in this case is not ethical in the strict sense but quasi-religious or spiritual, but I am not interested in driving a sharp wedge between the ethical and the religious or spiritual.

11. Habermas argues that genetic control violates autonomy and undermines the grounds of equality. See Habermas, *Future of Human Nature*. The problem with the first argument is that because the alternative to having one's genetic constitution chosen by one's parents is not choosing it oneself but having it given by nature, it is difficult to see where there is any violation of autonomy.

12. See Fukuyama, *Our Posthuman Future*, 49, 57; Kass, *Life, Liberty*, 122; and President's Council on Bioethics, *Beyond Therapy*, 85–94.

13. See Kass, *Toward a More Natural Science*, 157–86; and Sandel, *Case against Perfection*, 46–47.

14. A classic scenario involves two young boys who have the same projected adult height, one of whom suffers from human growth hormone deficiency, a recognized disease, and the other of whom simply has below-normal stature. Strictly adhered to, the therapy-enhancement distinction would seem to permit growth hormone treatment for the former but not the latter, even though both suffer the social disadvantages that often accompany low stature. A similar but not identical kind of case arises with the prospect of safe and effective memory-suppressing drugs. Those humanistic naturalists who would be willing to justify the use of such a drug to treat those who suffer from posttraumatic stress disorder (PTSD) would likely be troubled by the use of it to suppress unpleasant memories more generally. But the sufficient rationale for justifying the former use is not that PTSD is a disease while the other states in which unpleasant memories occur presumably are not, but rather that the memories activated in PTSD episodes are so disturbing that they cause acute suffering and inhibit one from going on with her life. However, other memories may have similar effects, albeit to lesser degrees. The

difference is one of magnitude, and that would make it difficult to justify restricting the drug to the treatment of PTSD.

15. For one discussion, see McKenny, "Human Enhancement Uses of Biotechnology," 507–15. Also see chapter 1 in this book.

16. See Nussbaum, "Transcending Humanity," 380–81.

17. Aquinas stresses the cooperation of natural human capacities with divine grace. It is possible, while still holding that divine grace cooperates with human capacities, to emphasize the sufficiency of grace in bringing about the communion of human beings with God and to think of the exercise of natural human capacities as a response, initiated and empowered by grace, to what grace has already accomplished. According to Barth, to be human is to be a creature whose relation to God is constituted from outside itself by grace, and therefore apart from its own natural capacities, but which, precisely as it is transcended from without in this way, is enabled to transcend itself outward as it responds to grace; see Barth, *Church Dogmatics, Volume III, Part 2,* 162–66. Grace, having already secured the relationship between humans and God which human beings are unable to secure by their powers, summons the human being to respond, and it is this summons that constitutes human beings as the creatures they are and distinguishes them from other creatures. Yet the response to grace, though empowered by grace, is nevertheless the exercise of a natural creaturely capacity. It is only by virtue of what transcends her from outside, namely grace, that the human creature is in a position to respond to God at all. Human beings do not have by nature the capability of maintaining their being in relation to God and can only misuse and corrupt their nature by ignoring the summons of grace. Yet in both cases—whether in affirming grace or rejecting it—one expresses one's human nature—by fulfilling its purpose in the first case and by contradicting it in the second case.

18. Aquinas, *Summa Theologica,* I.12.4, 5, 7. A complete account of Aquinas's position would also have to take account of the love of God that is ultimately inseparable from the knowledge of God, and therefore of the role of grace in extending human moral capacities.

19. This is a point that humanistic naturalist critics of external transcendence—who assume that any encounter with a transcendent good must come at the expense of our humanity—fail to grasp.

20. The claim that the ultimate good is one to be enjoyed by humans alone among creatures does not entail the claims that human capacities are superior to those of other creatures, that the only genuine goods are those to be enjoyed by humans, or even that other creatures—whether animals or posthumans—do not or would not enjoy some form of communion with God and thus participate in some way in the ultimate good. Christian theology permits and even demands the claim that all creation communes with God in some way. In any case, for Christian theology enjoyment of the ultimate good, though it requires having the capacities humans have, does not depend on those capacities being the most superior capacities of any creature. If technological enhancement does eventually result in something we may legitimately name "posthuman," it would simply give humans

one more reason for expressing the wonder of the Psalmist at God's regard for humanity: "What are human beings that you are mindful of them, mortals that you care for them?" (Ps 8:4).

21. Humanity+, "Transhumanist Declaration."

22. Humanity+, "Transhumanist FAQ."

23. Ibid.

24. Bostrom, "Transhumanist Values," 93.

25. Ibid., 95.

26. See Humanity+, "Transhumanist Declaration"; and Humanity+, "Transhumanist FAQ." The extraordinary naïveté of most transhumanists is not mitigated by their recognition that the transhumanist project could go horribly bad or by their sincere determination to put in place an ethical framework that would prevent a moral catastrophe. Their naïveté results from their failure to recognize that beings with different natural capacities than ours (even other human beings with significantly different capabilities) would not necessarily acknowledge their full moral solidarity with us and may even have radically different moral dispositions than we have, and that the modern moral framework on which they rely is powerless to restrain (and may well contribute to) the use of technology to form subjects in accordance with social norms in ways that far exceed what pre-technological methods can do. The former point was made well by Nietzsche and the latter by Foucault, but both are discussed at length by Fukuyama, *Our Postmodern Future*; and Sandel, *Case against Perfection*.

27. Of course, for Christians, too, the ultimate good is unknowable and always will be, even in its full enjoyment in eternity. However, the good is not entirely unknown, or unenjoyed, even in this life. Most important, it has been fully known and enjoyed in a fully human life by Jesus Christ and is ultimately enjoyed by us through our participation in Christ. Christian theology, so understood, avoids the dilemma of transcendence described by Hegel, according to which any experience of the transcendent renders it immanent, whereas anything transcendent that is not experienced is merely empty.

References

Aquinas, Thomas. *Summa Theologica*, translated by Fathers of the English Dominican Province. 5 vols. New York: Benziger Brothers, 1948.

Barth, Karl. *Church Dogmatics, Volume III, Part 2: The Doctrine of Creation*, translated by Harold Knight, G. W. Bromiley, J. K. S. Reid, and R. H. Fuller. Edinburgh: T. & T. Clark, 1960.

Bostrom, Nick. "Transhumanist Values." *Review of Contemporary Philosophy* 4 (2005): 87–101.

Fukuyama, Francis. *Our Posthuman Future: Consequences of the Biotechnological Revolution*. New York: Farrar, Straus & Giroux, 2002.

———. "The World's Most Dangerous Ideas: Transhumanism." *Foreign Policy* 144 (2004): 42–43.

Habermas, Jürgen. *The Future of Human Nature*. Cambridge: Polity Press, 2003.

Harris, John. *Enhancing Evolution: The Ethical Case for Making Better People.* Princeton, NJ: Princeton University Press, 2007.

———. *Wonderwoman and Superman: The Ethics of Human Biotechnology.* Oxford: Oxford University Press, 1992.

Humanity+, "Transhumanist Declaration." http://humanityplus.org/learn/transhumanist-declaration/.

———. "Transhumanist FAQ." http://humanityplus.org/learn/transhumanist-faq/.

Jonas, Hans. *The Imperative of Responsibility.* Chicago: University of Chicago Press, 1984.

Kass, Leon. *Life, Liberty, and the Pursuit of Dignity.* San Francisco: Encounter Books, 2003.

———. *Toward a More Natural Science.* New York: Free Press, 1985.

McKenny, Gerald P. "Human Enhancement Uses of Biotechnology, Ethics, Therapy vs. Enhancement." In *Encyclopedia of Ethical, Legal and Policy Issues in Biotechnology,* edited by Thomas Murray and Maxwell J. Mehlman. New York: John Wiley & Sons, 2000.

Nussbaum, Martha. "Transcending Humanity." Reprinted as chapter 15 of *Love's Knowledge,* by Martha Nussbaum. New York: Oxford University Press, 1990.

President's Council on Bioethics, ed. *Beyond Therapy: Biotechnology and the Pursuit of Happiness.* New York: HarperCollins, 2003. http://bioethics.georgetown.edu/pcbe/reports/beyondtherapy/beyond_therapy_final_webcorrected.pdf.

Sandel, Michael. *The Case against Perfection: Ethics in the Age of Genetic Engineering.* Cambridge, MA: Harvard University Press, 2007.

Taylor, Charles. "Review Article on Martha Nussbaum: The Fragility of Goodness—Luck and Ethics in Greek Tragedy and Philosophy." *Canadian Journal of Philosophy* 18 (1998): 805–14.

———. *A Secular Age.* Cambridge, MA: Harvard University Press, 2007.

Chapter Thirteen

Transhumanism and Christianity

RONALD COLE-TURNER

The scholars who contributed to this book hold differing views on transhumanism and on the use of technology for human enhancement. Even so, several shared themes and common perspectives are clearly visible. For example, the contributors generally recognize that on the surface, at least, there are notable similarities between Christianity and transhumanism. Christians hope for eternal life that will be enjoyed with the fullest possible knowledge, joy, and moral purity. Transhumanists look forward to extending the human life span perhaps indefinitely while also enriching human knowledge, attaining greater happiness if not joy, and achieving moral balance or social harmony. One explanation of these similarities is that transhumanism has emerged from a culture shaped by Christianity. Another is that the yearnings of Christians and transhumanists, if not quite universally shared by all human beings, are broadly held and find their own expression in both contexts and perhaps elsewhere.

The contributors agree that transhumanism presents a new challenge for theology and for the lives of ordinary Christians. How should Christians today view the emerging technologies of human enhancement? In light of these technologies, how should they view salvation? Some Christians may respond by trying to avoid enhancement technology altogether, holding to divine grace as the only valid pathway to true human fulfillment and transformation. Others may think that technology seems to provide something remarkably like what the Christian faith promises and therefore replaces the need for faith. Still others might find a way to enfold the limited enhancements of technology into the fuller transformations of faith.

In fairness it needs to be noted that the contributors all agree with transhumanism on one important assumption, which is based on a shared acceptance of the theory of evolution as the best explanation of diversity and change in living organisms. Thus the contributors all accept the transhumanist starting point that biological organisms, including human beings, are evolved, changing, and possibly changeable, perhaps even through technological intervention. Human nature as it exists today was not created in its present form. Of course, we could find other theologians who would argue for a creationist view and who would object to transhumanism on the basis that human nature should be seen as fixed and final and that it is either impossible or inherently immoral to try to change it. We have not taken that course here, first because we think it is theologically questionable to dismiss the well-verified findings of science, but more so because the focus of our attention is on theology and technology and not on theology and evolution.

Shared Criticisms of Transhumanism

The contributors to this book also agree that from the perspective of Christian theology, transhumanism is open to several criticisms. Though the argument is not explicitly developed in the preceding chapters, nearly every Christian theologian agrees that technologies of human enhancement pose a new challenge for anyone concerned about social and economic justice. The concern is not simply that the wealthy may be able to buy something that the poor cannot afford, but also that by purchasing enhancement technology, the wealthy might in turn convert their present wealth into future power, thereby widening the social gap between the few who are enhanced and the many who remain merely natural. This is especially worrisome if technology actually does succeed in engineering a new, posthuman species.[1]

Some of the chapters above, especially chapter 7 by J. Jeanine Thweatt-Bates and chapter 8 by Celia Deane-Drummond, object to the transhumanist desire to escape the limitations of biology, which can only be seen as the latest form of the desire to flee the body. The contributors all tend to argue that transhumanists hold a view of the human self that is characterized by some of the Enlightenment's more questionable assumptions, in particular the view of the self as a disembodied center of consciousness and will that uses technology to control the body and the environment but somehow remains largely unaffected by either. The most extreme version of disembodiment in transhumanism thinking, as Brent Waters points out in chapter 11, is found in the suggestion by Hans Moravec and Ray Kurzweil that the human self might escape death by uploading a digital version of the sum total of the mental life into one or more computers, there to live on as if little else has changed. In somewhat less extreme forms, a tendency toward a disembodied view of the self runs through many parts of the transhumanist movement.

Another theological criticism of transhumanism, made explicit in chapter 5 by Ted Peters, is that transhumanists seem a little naive about the human predicament and therefore overly optimistic about what it takes to engineer solutions. What theologians call "sin"—humanity's unexplained but inescapable tendency to pervert and destroy even its best achievements—is missing from transhumanist thought, and also absent is any realistic attitude about how well and, at the same time, how badly things will go as we make "progress" toward improving our lives and our species. Our technological power is great and it is growing quickly, but it is never pure, never character-ized by singularity of purpose in pursuit of the good. If this self-sabotaging inner disorder is a "limitation of our biology," it is one that we seem unable or unwilling to transcend, all the more so because too rarely do we admit that it is real.

Theological Disagreements

Although generally agreeing on the points noted above, the contributors to this volume disagree among themselves about the most appropriate Christian response to transhumanism. Their disagreements seem to center on this question: Just how far should human beings take the task of their own improvement into their own hands, using not just the moral and spiri-tual disciplines of the religious life but also such things as technology? To what extent are we to accept the world as given, limiting our expectations and our interventions? Many people today believe that we need to learn to say "enough," to stop before we go too far or destroy too much. To what degree should we accept our human frailties and limits without meddling and complaining? Or conversely, to what extent are we to embrace our strengths, including our power and our duty to improve ourselves and our world? When should we see disease, a lack of resources, and unmet longings as challenges that can and should be addressed by all our means, including technology? This disagreement is not likely to go away, perhaps because it runs deeper than theology and only manifests itself here in a particularly theological way.

In a recent essay that probes below the surface of the secular debate about the use of technology for human enhancement, Erik Parens distinguishes between two frames of mind, two conflicting but equally valid attitudes that are reflected in the debate. He identifies these as "the gratitude or creativity framework."[2] In many respects, he suggests, the current debate is driven by a conflict between these two frameworks: "As one side emphasizes our obliga-tion to remember that life is a gift and that we need to learn to let things be, the other emphasizes our obligation to transform that gift and to exhibit our creativity."[3] What is too often overlooked, he suggests, is that most thought-ful people recognize that the truth can be found in both frameworks: "Most of us can be comfortable in both frameworks, even if most of us are consid-erably more comfortable in one framework than in the other. I should hurry to add: Moving between frameworks, being ambivalent, seems to me to be a sign of openness and thoughtfulness, not confusion."[4]

Not only does Parens recognize the religious sources of both frameworks, but he is also clear to point out that neither one is decidedly religious or notably secular. In comparing Christians and secular thinkers, for example, some might think that Christians take the position of gratitude while the secularists take the side of creativity. What Parens helps us see is "the religious element of the commitments on both sides."[5] The difference between the two frameworks is not the same "as the difference between people who are religious and those who are secular. You find both kinds in both camps."[6] This is certainly true of the contributors to this volume, who agree on many matters of theology but disagree on how much they sympathize with the core transhumanist notion that technology can truly enhance human life. Parens's description of the conflict between the frameworks of gratitude and creativity is one way to understand the different perspectives expressed in this book.

More profoundly, however, the conflict between frameworks is something that runs right through the views of each contributor to this volume, which seem to always recognize the truth found in both "gratitude" and "creativity." In their own way, each author seems to recognize the truth of what Waters calls "remaining creaturely" in chapter 11, and, at the same time, are in accord with Michael Spezio's appeal in chapter 10 for a theology that affirms human maturity and creativity, not frailty and passivity. If Parens is right, then the disagreement among the contributors is not surprising; nor is it likely to go away. It represents a productive and widely felt tension between two compelling points of view.

We might note finally that the gratitude / creativity tension is something that Christian theology tends to locate in the very nature of God—and thus we might perhaps now rename the frameworks as "blessing" and "re-creation" rather than gratitude and creativity. For Christians, God expresses both frameworks, as the Creator who redeems and transforms. In Genesis 1, God pronounces the creation good, and then in the rest of the Bible the same God seeks its redemption and transformation. The God who created is also the one who "makes all things new."[7] When Christian theologians find themselves drawn to both of Parens's frameworks, it is because they see this polarity as foundational not just to their view of humanity but also of the God in whose image we are created.

Salvation and Transformation in an Age of Technology

Chapter 1 of this book began by asking: Who is in a position to judge whether an "enhancement" really is an improvement? We saw that, according to

Maxwell Mehlman, the answer is that "for the most part, an enhancement is an improvement if the enhanced person thinks it is one."[8] Chapter 1 went on to point out a problem with this answer. What if the "enhancement" is effective in changing the brain and the perspective of the enhanced person, who now sees the "enhancement" not as an improvement but as the opposite? Which person—preenhancement or postenhancement—correctly judges whether the enhancement really enhances? Precisely because an enhancement might change the embodied self or the embodied will, it changes the referee.

Leaving the decision about what counts as an enhancement up to the modified individual may be the only way a pluralistic society can avoid a new source of conflict. For the Christian, however, the decision about what counts as an enhancement is not based on personal preference but on accepting the truth that our lives are already being transformed in what must be called "salvation." Our true enhancement is not defined by individual preference but by the standard of what God is doing to transform us. Though the individual Christian must consent to salvation, individuals are never consulted about where it takes us or what it means to be saved. Salvation, as we shall see, is expressly *not* the fulfillment of our desires for ourselves. It is the replacement of our desire for the self with a desire for God.

One of the problems facing theology today is that it is not as clear as it should be about how to understand salvation. Too often in popular Christianity, salvation is an empty placeholder, preached as necessary but left open to just about any interpretation or expectation, including too many that are not shaped as much by scripture or Christian tradition as by social and cultural trends. Long before the arrival of enhancement technology, Christians too frequently allowed their understanding of salvation to be distorted so that it became a self-enhancement program, a personal benefits package that requires nothing. If Christianity is to offer a real critique of the culture of enhancement technology, its foundation must stand apart from this culture and be based on something quite different, something rooted in the core of Christian theology and its distinctive view of salvation through Christ. By claiming that the validity of any enhancement must be judged in reference to salvation, Christian theology is saying that its view of the human condition and its amelioration is based on what scripture and tradition have to say about what God is doing to transform us. This topic, of course, is far beyond our scope, but three key points can be noted briefly.

First, the gift of salvation is made possible by the action of God in Jesus Christ, who assumes our human condition as necessary for the work of salvation. The Creator is the Savior, blessing and transforming at one and the same time. For this reason, Christians recognize the continuity of creation and redemption, not as the contrary actions of rival gods or even as two chapters in the actions of one God, but as one continuous action of creation and transformation, often aptly called "the new creation." We are not saved from the world, either through disembodiment or escape from destruction, but in and with the transformation of the whole creation. Furthermore, the Creator is the Savior *incarnate*. The creation is not saved apart from human involvement, as if by divine action from a distance, for it is only in the humanity of the incarnate Christ that God acts to save the world. For Christian theology, the entire sweep of incarnate creation–transformation is one unbroken work of God, inclusive of all that we have now come to see as the history and future of the cosmos. The incarnate Creator is the Redeemer. Just as the work of creation is not divided from redemption, the work of God is joined with the action of creation by virtue of the Incarnation.

On this basis, Christianity should not separate creation and redemption, nor should it divide the work of God from the action of the creature. In chapter 5 Ted Peters quotes the Lutheran theologian Carl Braaten on the distinction between futurology and eschatology: "A crucial difference between secular futurology and Christian eschatology is this: The future in secular futurology is *reached* by a process of the world's *becoming*. The future in Christian eschatology *arrives* by the *coming* of God's kingdom. The one is a *becoming* and the other a *coming*."[9] Clearly we can distinguish between becoming and arriving, between creation's achievement and God's gift. But on the basis of the Incarnation, the two cannot be separated. For this reason, theology cannot dismiss technology or even set it aside as if it were not part of the whole incarnate creative and redemptive work of God.

Second, for Christianity, the pathway of salvation begins with an act of renunciation, what scripture often calls "repentance," which is a turning away from our old ways even if they are not particularly evil but just because they are our own. Repentance is not a rejection of creation but of willful disobedience and self-centered thinking. It is the simple recognition that to enter the new, we must let go of the old. We are to let go of our "old life" in order to enter into a new kind of life, ordered not by our own plans or desires but by those exemplified in Jesus Christ, who wholly gives himself to the will of God in service of others. The paradox at the heart of Christianity is that by losing our lives, we gain true life. This is perhaps the sharpest point of divergence between Christianity and transhumanism.

On the basis of this difference, Christian theology is driven to make a criticism of transhumanism that is difficult to state with subtlety or graciousness. But it must be said that according to Christian theology, transhumanists seem both human-centered and self-centered, concerned chiefly with humanity above other species and with themselves among other humans. Is it not the case that the central concern of the transhumanist is the enhancement of the self? Here again, perhaps we are in their debt for making explicit what is often unsaid about the whole enterprise of enhancement technology—that it is absorbed with the self and its preservation and expansion. It must be said most emphatically that Christians do not claim to be less selfish or better people than anyone, merely that they admit this fact about themselves as a failing rather than affirm it as the basis for a social movement. And for this reason Christians must object, even if it is with more than a tinge of hypocrisy, to what they see as the self-aggrandizing, self-expanding tendency that drives transhumanism.

For Christianity, the place to start is with self-emptying, not self-fulfillment. Though it is true that Christian theology strongly affirms the transformation and glorification of the cosmos and of the human creature, we must be wary of focusing our attention only on this point, particularly at the expense of the requirement that the path to glorification lies through renunciation. If we were to make this mistake, we could easily come to the erroneous conclusion that Christianity and transhumanism are in fundamental agreement. If Christians and transhumanists share similar hopes, they expressly do not share the same assumptions about the precondition of renunciation of the self. Christians will always suspect that transhumanists are essentially egocentric. Christians may be just as self-centered, but at least they know that they are supposed to recognize their self-centeredness as a sin standing in the way of their true enhancement.

Third, with the requirement of renunciation clearly in mind, it is also true that traditional Christianity sees salvation in the most transformative terms possible. The renunciation of willfulness is never a repudiation of the creation or the creature. On the contrary, the end of salvation is the glorification of the whole creation centered on the human creature, transformed and exalted far beyond anything that transhumanism envisions. Salvation is not just rescue or restoration, although it must be acknowledged that too often Western Christianity has reduced salvation to little more than the forgiveness of sins and the restoration of humanity's relationship with God, essentially resetting the moral clock to the time of Adam and Eve before the Fall.

At this point the parallel between the therapy/enhancement distinction and the restoration/glorification contrast, noted briefly in chapter 1, comes to mind once again. Although the Western Church (including Protestantism) has generally limited salvation to restoration or "therapy," the early church and the theologians of Eastern Orthodoxy today more correctly see salvation as exaltation and glorification that goes far beyond the enhancement hopes of transhumanism. Salvation is a process of transformation, an ontological change that makes it possible for the redeemed to participate eternally in the very life of God, not as disembodied or "uploaded" souls but as transformed beings in a transfigured creation. On the basis of this belief, Christians will see transhumanism as too limited.

The Greek term *theosis*, introduced in chapter 9 by Todd Daly, is sometimes used to describe the process of transformation, but originally the idea was seen as too extreme by Western theologians, who have avoided the term until recently. What the term implies is that God is transforming human beings to such an extent that God is making us "godlike." The transformation is both moral and ontological. Through *theosis*, the believer is progressively being made holy, conforming not to the values of the age but to the virtues of the Christian life, exemplified by Christ. But the believer is also being made a new creature, in the end a new kind of glorified being who will enjoy what might be described as youthful health, fullness of knowledge, and immortality. On the basis of this view of salvation as *theosis*, it can be said that Christian theology finds fault with transhumanism not because it says that human beings should be enhanced but because it holds too limited a view of human transformation.

Theology, Technology, and the Future

Transhumanism, however, presents a challenge of its own for Christianity. The transhumanist might ask: "If Christianity is in favor of transformation, and seemingly without limits, is it also in favor of the use of technology as a means of transformation? Do you Christians merely wait passively to be saved, or are you willing—as Pierre Teilhard de Chardin maintains and as the Bible itself says—to 'work out your own salvation'?"[10]

How will Christian theology answer the transhumanist's question about the appropriate role of technology in helping to bring about the transformation of the creation and of human beings? Theological ideas about technology go back to the earliest church, whose theologians interpreted biblical texts about creation in the light of philosophy and current technology, reaching the conclusion that God intended for human beings to develop and use technology. From the Greek philosophers, they borrowed the idea that in comparison with all other animals, human beings are unprepared to survive except by their wits and inventions. Lacking claws, we were forced to make knives and spears, and so forth. Theologians saw this not as a deficit but as a planned incentive. God created us unprepared in order to force us to invent.

In recent decades, however, theologians have been more cautious about technology. The French Reformed theologian Jacques Ellul (1912–94) was critical not just of the misuses of technology but also of the way in which it transforms our thinking. Even those theologians who are largely supportive of technology recognize that it can be used to cause great harm. Thus Teilhard de Chardin, whose views are presented in chapters 2 and 3, takes an unusually optimistic view that technology is the means whereby the creation will reach its next stage and that any problems will be more than worked out in the end. Without technology, Teilhard believed, the creative purposes of God would be stopped or at least dramatically slowed.

Even if Teilhard is too optimistic and Ellul is too alarmist, theology today can and must reflect on the issues they raised and on the growing power of technology since their time. The creativity and scope of technology must be acknowledged for the way in which it changes both the social and the natural reality that theology faces. At the same time theologians must remain clear about the disappointments and dangers posed by technology. A key part of the challenge facing theology, however, is to keep technology from so completely changing the way we see the world that we lose the richer, more embodied, more emotional and complicated meaning of our human relationships, our yearnings, our failures, and our attempts to begin anew. The point is not that we need to lean on God because we are weak but that we need to engage in a relationship with God all the more because we are strong and growing stronger. We need to be aware that technology, precisely because of its beneficial power, can lead us to the erroneous notion that the only problems to which it is worth paying attention involve engineering. When we let this happen, we reduce human yearning for salvation to a mere desire for enhancement, a lesser salvation that we can control rather than the true salvation for which we must also wait.

Saying that we must wait for the true salvation does not imply, however, that technology has no role to play, just that technology plays only a part. Too often, secular advocates of technology think that Christian theologians are opposed to technology because it threatens God's prerogatives over creation. It must be admitted that some theologians sometimes write as if they believe this. But as a general rule, it is simply not true that theology rejects technology because it limits God, or even that theology rejects technology at all. Theology's main concern with technology is the way human beings claim it as their own and use it only for what they suppose is human benefit. For the Christian, technology may be powerful, but it is not ours. It is God's, and its purpose is to expand the ways in which God's work can be done.

Such a view of technology is suggested by the twentieth-century Romanian theologian Dumitru Stăniloae: "The human person . . . has his own part in creating himself; he is not created by God only. And, in part, the human person also creates the world. He can freely bring into act some or other of the potentialities of the world, and because God assists man toward this end, God himself remains in relationship of freedom to the world and in a relationship of free collaboration with the human person."[11] The human role is critically important for Stăniloae, as long as it is not seen as autonomous. "The Spirit is also at work through the incarnate spirit, which is our own being. In this way the working of the human person, made strong by the power of God, is at one and the same time an activity of the human person and of God, a synergic operation. Indeed, synergy is the general formula for the working of God in the world."[12]

What the Christian is not prepared to do, however, is to assume that human beings are sufficiently wise or good to be trusted to guide the process whereby technology affects the future of evolution—if indeed it does. Transhumanists seem willing to take this risk. Evolution, for all its creativity, is morally neutral or blind. According to transhumanism, human beings are rational and moral and are therefore equipped, not just technologically but also morally, to direct evolution's next step.

The transhumanist view is stated by Julian Savulescu: "The next stage of human evolution will be rational evolution, where we select children who not only have the greatest chance of surviving, reproducing and being free of disease, but who have the greatest opportunities to have the best lives in their likely environment. Evolution was indifferent to how well our lives went. We are not."[13] It is not that Christians think that evolution has our best interests "in mind." On this point, there is no disagreement with the transhumanist. The disagreement is about whether human beings truly have their own best interests in mind. For the transhumanist, if not human beings, then who else knows what is good for us? For the Christian, what is good for human beings is what truly transcends us and raises us to an unexpected exaltation.

Notes

1. For more on enhancement and justice, see Cole-Turner, "Religion, Genetics, and the Future," 201–23.

2. Parens, "Toward a More Fruitful Debate," 189.

3. Ibid.

4. Ibid.

5. Ibid., 190.

6. Ibid., 191.

7. Rev 21:5: "And the one who was seated on the throne said, 'See, I am making all things new'" (NRSV).

8. Mehlman, *Price of Perfection*, 6.

9. Braaten, *Future of God*, 29.

10. Phil 2:12–13: "Therefore, my beloved, just as you have always obeyed me, not only in my presence, but much more now in my absence, work out your own

salvation with fear and trembling; for it is God who is at work in you, enabling you both to will and to work for his good pleasure" (NRSV).

11. Stăniloae, *Experience of God*, 44.

12. Ibid., 60–61.

13. Savulescu, "Genetic Interventions," 13; cf. Bostrom and Sandberg, "Wisdom of Nature," 375–416.

References

Bostrom, Nick, and Anders Sandberg. "The Wisdom of Nature: An Evolutionary Heuristic for Human Enhancement." In *Human Enhancement*, edited by Julian Savulescu and Nick Bostrom. New York: Oxford University Press, 2009.

Braaten, Carl E. *The Future of God*. New York: Harper & Row, 1969.

Cole-Turner, Ronald. "Religion, Genetics, and the Future." In *Design and Destiny: Jewish and Christian Perspectives on Human Germline Modification*, edited by Ronald Cole-Turner. Cambridge, MA: MIT Press, 2008.

Mehlman, Maxwell J. *The Price of Perfection: Individualism and Society in the Era of Biomedical Enhancement*. Baltimore: Johns Hopkins University Press, 2009.

Parens, Erik. "Toward a More Fruitful Debate about Enhancement." In *Human Enhancement*, edited by Nick Bostrom and Anders Sandberg. New York: Oxford University Press, 2009.

Savulescu, Julian. "Genetic Interventions and the Ethics of Enhancement of Human Beings." Available at www.abc.net.au/rn/backgroundbriefing/documents/savulescu_chapter.pdf

Stăniloae, Dumitru. *The Experience of God: Orthodox Dogmatic Theology, Volume 2—The World: Creation and Deification*, translated by Ioan Ionita and Robert Barringer. Brookline, MA: Holy Cross Orthodox Press, 2000.

Contributors

Michael Burdett is a DPhil candidate in theology at the University of Oxford (Regents Park College). He received degrees in engineering, physics, and theology, and he has been given academic and professional awards in each field and has worked as a systems engineer for the Northrop Grumman Corporation. Currently, he is a student at the Oxford Centre for Christianity and Culture, where his research focuses on continental philosophy, the technological society, and Christian theology. His dissertation is titled "The God of Possibility and Promise: Christian Eschatology in Response to Technological Futurism."

Ronald Cole-Turner holds the H. Parker Sharp Chair in Theology and Ethics at Pittsburgh Theological Seminary, a position devoted to exploring the implications of science and technology for Christian theology and ethics. He previously taught at Memphis Theological Seminary and is a graduate of Princeton Theological Seminary. His most recent book is *Design and Destiny: Jewish and Christian Theological Perspectives on Human Germline Modification* (MIT Press, 2008).

Todd T. W. Daly is assistant professor of theology and ethics at Urbana Theological Seminary. He holds a PhD from the University of Edinburgh in systematic theology. He is author of "Life-Extension in Transhumanist and Christian Perspectives: Consonance and Conflict," *Journal of Evolution and Technology* (2005). He is currently writing a book that explores the ethical implications that arise from the medical prolongation of life and aging. Portions of this work have appeared in *Christianity Today* and *Touchstone: A Journal of Mere Christianity*. His research interests include theological ethics, *theosis*, the moral force of embodiment, enhancement technologies, and the uses of scripture in Christian ethics.

Celia Deane-Drummond holds a chair in theology and the biological sciences at the University of Chester, where she serves as director of the Centre for Religion and the Biosciences. She is vice chair of the European Forum for the Study of Religion and Environment and editor of a book series titled *Re-Visioning Ethics* (SCM Press). She holds degrees and doctorates in the natural science (Cambridge University and Reading University) and theology (Council for National Academic Awards and Manchester University). She has published more than thirty scientific articles, numerous articles and chapters in theology and ethics, and more than fifteen books in different areas connecting theology or ethics with science. Her recent books include *Brave New World* (2003, edited), *Re-Ordering Nature* (2003, coedited), *The Ethics of Nature* (2004), *Future Perfect* (2006, coedited), *Genetics and Christian Ethics* (2006), *Ecotheology* (2008), *Christ and Evolution* (2009), *Creaturely Theology* (2009, coedited), and *Religion and Ecology in the Public Sphere* (2011, coedited).

Stephen Garner is lecturer in practical theology in the School of Theology at the University of Auckland. He holds an MSc in computer science and a PhD in theology. He has worked in a variety of information technology fields, including software engineering, machine learning research, and e-learning. He currently teaches in the areas of theological ethics, public and contextual theology, science and religion, religion and popular culture, and spirituality. His research interests focus on the interaction of technology, theology, and popular culture, and his PhD dissertation is titled "Transhumanism and the *Imago Dei*: Narratives of Apprehension and Hope." He is also a member of the New Zealand Interchurch Bioethics Council, representing the Presbyterian Church of Aotearoa New Zealand.

David Grumett is research fellow in theology at the University of Exeter. He has published widely on modern French Catholic theology, including *Teilhard de Chardin: Theology, Humanity and Cosmos* (Peeters, 2005), *De Lubac: A Guide for the Perplexed* (T. & T. Clark, 2007), and articles on Maurice Blondel and Yves de Montcheuil. Building on this research, he is currently developing a constructive theological account of materiality by viewing eucharistic substance as exemplary of general substance. He also has interests in theology and material practice, having produced, with Rachel Muers, *Theology on the Menu: Asceticism, Meat and Christian Diet* (Routledge, 2010); and *Eating and Believing: Interdisciplinary Essays on Vegetarianism and Theology* (T. & T. Clark, 2008).

Karen Lebacqz served on the Pacific School of Religion faculty in the Graduate Theological Union for more than thirty years. Her lifelong commitment to issues of social justice takes shape in three primary areas of writing and teaching: professional ethics, bioethics (especially questions about genetics and the Human Genome Project), and ethical theory (particularly justice and questions of method in ethics). Her publications include a number of books, among them *Justice in an Unjust World*, *Sex in the Parish*, and *Sacred Cells? Why Christians Should Support Stem Cell Research*, coauthored with Ted Peters and Gaymon Bennett (2008). Her dozens of essays in bioethics, feminist ethics, and sexual ethics have been published in scientific journals, church magazines, and international contexts.

Gerald McKenny is Walter Professor of Theology at the University of Notre Dame. He is the author of *The Analogy of Grace: Karl Barth's Moral Theology* (2010) and *To Relieve the Human Condition* (1997). He has coedited *Altering Nature* (2 volumes, 2008) and *The Ethical* (2002), a volume of essays on continental moral philosophy. He has published widely in the fields of Christian ethics and biomedical ethics and is writing a book on Christian ethics and biotechnology.

Ted Peters is professor of systematic theology at Pacific Lutheran Theological Seminary and the Graduate Theological Union in Berkeley, California. He serves as coeditor of the journal *Theology and Science*, published by the Center for Theology and the Natural Sciences. He is author of *God: The World's Future* (Fortress Press, rev. ed.,

2000); *Playing God? Genetic Determinism and Human Freedom* (Routledge, rev. ed., 2003); *Science, Theology, and Ethics* (Ashgate, 2003); and *Anticipating Omega* (Vandenhoeck & Ruprecht, 2007). He is coauthor of *Sacred Cells? Why Christians Should Support Stem Cell Research*, with Karen Lebacqz and Gaymon Bennett (2008); *Can You Believe in God and Evolution?* (Abingdon Press, 2006); and coeditor of *Bridging Science and Religion* (Fortress, 2002).

Michael L. Spezio, an assistant professor of psychology and neuroscience at Scripps College, is a social neuroscientist who seeks to understand the systems of the mind and brain that underlie evaluative cognition, specifically in the social domain. He received his MDiv from Pittsburgh Theological Seminary and his PhD in cognitive/ systems neuroscience from the University of Oregon. He is coeditor of two forthcoming volumes, *The Routledge Companion to Religion & Science* and *Theology and the Science of Morality: Virtue Ethics, Exemplarity, and Cognitive Neuroscience*. He has recently published papers on social neuroscience in the *American Economic Review*, *Social Cognitive and Affective Neuroscience*, and the *Journal of Neuroscience*. He is a member of the International Society for Science and Religion and continues to investigate the cognitive and neural processes of social decision making, with a focus on autism, political judgment, and empathy and compassion in morally relevant action, and the role of contemplative practices in reshaping these processes. He is also an ordained minister of the Presbyterian Church (USA).

J. Jeanine Thweatt-Bates holds a PhD from Princeton Theological Seminary in theology and science. She is the author of *Cyborg Selves: A Theological Anthropology of the Posthuman* (Ashgate, in press) and currently serves as an instructor at the Science for Ministry Institute in Princeton, New Jersey. Her research focuses on the intersection of feminism, theology, and science and on the issues of technology and embodiment.

Brent Waters is Jerre and Mary Joy Stead Professor of Christian Social Ethics at Garrett-Evangelical Theological Seminary, where he also directs the Jerre L. and Mary Joy Stead Center for Ethics and Values. He is the author of *Economic Globalization and Christian Ethics* (in press) and *Christian Moral Theology in an Emerging Technoculture* (in press). His recent publications include *This Mortal Flesh: Incarnation and Bioethics* (2009); *The Family in Christian Social and Political Thought* (2007); and *From Human to Posthuman: Christian Theology and Technology in a Postmodern World* (2006). He also serves on the advisory board of *Christian Bioethics*. He received his DPhil from the University of Oxford.

Index